The Diet Detect...

ALL-AMERICAN DIET

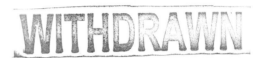

Also by Charles Platkin

Breaking the Pattern

Breaking the Fat Pattern / The Automatic Diet

Lighten Up

The Diet Detective's Count Down

The Diet Detective's Calorie Bargain Bible

The Diet Detective's

ALL-AMERICAN DIET

Take Control of Your Diet
and Eat the Foods You Already Love and Want

The Alternative to Jenny Craig® *or* NutriSystem®

Thousands of Easy-to-Use Mix-and-Match "Build-a-Meals"
from Your Favorite Supermarket and Restaurant Foods

Charles Platkin, PhD

RODALE

© 2012 by Charles Platkin, PhD

All rights reserved. No part of this publication may be reproduced or transmitted in any form or by any means, electronic or mechanical, including photocopying, recording, or any other information storage and retrieval system, without the written permission of the publisher.

Rodale books may be purchased for business or promotional use or for special sales. For information, please write to: Special Markets Department, Rodale Inc., 733 Third Avenue, New York, NY 10017.

Printed in the United States of America
Rodale Inc. makes every effort to use acid-free ∞, recycled paper ✿.

Book design by C. Linda Dingler

Library of Congress Cataloging-in-Publication Data is on file with the publisher.
ISBN-10: 1–60961–156–X paperback
ISBN-13: 978–1–60961–156–9

Distributed to the trade by Macmillan

2 4 6 8 10 9 7 5 3 1 paperback

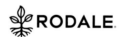

We inspire and enable people to improve their lives and the world around them.

www.rodalebooks.com

To my daughter, Parker South,
a constant inspiration, teacher, and joy;
to my parents, Linda and Norton,
who have always been and continue to be
a driving force in my life, as well as my biggest fans;
and to my wife, Shannon,
a patient, considerate, caring, and loving friend.

Contents

Build-a-Meal Foods

DINNER ENTRÉES (350–600 CALORIES)
(Choose One According to Your Plan)

DINNER SIDES (50–250 CALORIES)
(Choose One or More According to Your Plan)

FRUITS AND VEGETABLES (10–280 CALORIES)
(Choose According to Your Plan)

CONDIMENTS
(Each Counts as a Side)

Phase Three:
Maintain Your Weight Loss

Introduction

When people begin the process of weight control—or any behavior change, for that matter—they often wonder if they have enough willpower to actually make the change. Willpower is more or less about self-control, but simply knowing that resisting a piece of cake now (immediate gratification) will help you be trimmer, fitter, and healthier in the future (the long-term greater benefit) doesn't seem to cut it. As one researcher explained: A person standing right in front of you may seem larger (short-term reward) than a 70-story building in the distance (long-term greater reward). So the question is, do you need willpower to lose weight and get in shape, or is it something else?

Honestly, are you fond of stomping your foot on the kitchen floor, saying, "This is the last time! This is the last summer I'm going to be fat. I will lose the weight! I'm going to empty the refrigerator, clean out my cupboards, and never, ever eat junk food again"? The truth is that, more often than not, this approach is both extremely unpleasant and a big waste of energy. Do you really believe that all you need is a good, healthy dose of drawing a line in the sand to break the patterns you've been living by?

Look, I'm not going to sit here and tell you that there isn't some self-control or willpower involved in weight control, but it's significantly less than you think.

Losing and controlling weight appears to be *only* about willpower, but really it's about the preparation, the practice, the failure, the planning, and so on. Weight loss is more about power than willpower. You need to give yourself the power to lose weight.

The point is to not get discouraged because you think you lack the willpower or discipline to lose weight. That's not what's going to get you through this process.

Weight loss or control is not as simple as willing yourself not to eat that cookie. What *will* work is preparation and being honest with yourself about your behaviors. If there are particular cues or triggers that cause you to overeat, try to arrange your environment so that you avoid them as much as possible. So, for example, if the aroma wafting from the Dunkin' Donuts you pass each morning on your way to work draws you in like a magnet, change your route so that you aren't tempted.

By creating new routines for yourself, you will be making your new behaviors automatic. As I've said time and time again, it's just too difficult to think constantly about dieting—it will not work. Successful maintainers have figured out ways to make their behaviors and choices second nature. Activities like setting your alarm clock at night, putting on your shoes before leaving the house, and remembering how to drive to work do not require much thought. The idea is to apply the same principles to your diet.

For a long time, I've loved the concept of using frozen dinners, soups, cereals, and even restaurant foods to help people lose weight. Here's why: In the years I've spent helping people lose weight through counseling, working to change food policy, and trying to come up with methods for improving eating behaviors on a mass scale, I've learned something very valuable: It's hard enough to change *one* single behavior, let alone three, four, or even just two.

I can already hear the chatter from nutrition and health critics. "How can you recommend that people eat frozen foods? Fast foods? Oh my gosh! You have a PhD in public health, and *this* is what you're advising people to do?"

Point well taken. This is *not* a "grow your own organic garden, milk your own cow, raise your own chickens" type of diet. That's for sure.

The foods you'll find in *The Diet Detective's All-American Diet* are stepping-stones. You may not be able to go to the farmers' market on a daily basis and pick up organic produce. However, by using this book, you will lose weight, get more interested in fitness, gradually change your diet, and start living a brand-new life.

I know that's what happened for me. When I first lost my extra 50-plus pounds, my diet was to eat anything labeled "diet." I would have eaten a napkin if it had been labeled with the word *diet* and tasted okay.

Over time, I began to eat differently. Today I eat frozen foods, and I eat at restaurants, but my eating and exercise behaviors have moved to a new level so that I no longer have to follow as strict a plan. And so will yours over time.

The plan I've laid out is a wonderful first step. If you follow it, you *will* lose weight. The question is: *Can* you follow it? The answer is yes, because I've designed it specifically so that you will not be hungry. And you will not have to rely on chance or your own judgment to make good decisions about what to eat. All you have to do is choose from a wonderful variety of foods that you already know and follow the plan.

The Diet Detective's All-American Diet provides thousands of choices that allow you to create and build your very own daily menus using frozen foods (including organic options), ready-to-eat foods (e.g., soups, cereals, canned foods, fresh fruits, and vegetables), and foods available at the local supermarket, casual dining restaurants, fast-food chains, and even the local convenience store.

The best part? It's simple and requires virtually no cooking. *The Diet Detective's All-American Diet's* mix-and-match Build-a-Meal program shows you how to pick breakfast, lunch, dinner, and snack foods from lists of *thousands of popular, brand-name foods* available anywhere. You can actually use the lists no matter what diet you might currently be following. For instance, if you're on a 1,600-calorie program, just go to the 1,600-calorie meal plan on page 42, choose your meals based on those lists—and you'll be all set.

You can take these first steps and lose weight for good. I'm excited for you to get started. And congratulations! You've finally found something that will truly work for you.

It's just that simple.

Charles Platkin, PhD
New York City

PHASE ONE:

Getting Started

How and Why the Diet Detective's All-American Diet Works

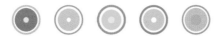

Most diets ask you to alter who you are and how you live. Well, that's not easy to do, particularly when it comes to eating behaviors. Most people go right back to their "comfort zones" when they encounter even a little bit of stress (kids screaming, a bad day at work, a traffic jam, etc.). Diets that ask you to eat a French or Mediterranean diet or eat like the Japanese are bound to fail.

The fact is you are *not* French, Mediterranean, or Japanese; you are American—that's your culture—and there's no reason to apologize or feel guilty about it. Americans eat foods that are easy, fast, and accessible.

Would it be healthier if you grew your own organic produce in your backyard garden? Of course. And doesn't going to the local farmers' market and buying foods to prepare for the evening's meal sound romantic and exciting? Certainly. But that way of life just isn't a reality for most Americans. Most Americans simply don't have the time to stand in the kitchen for 2 hours every day. Sure, we can learn from other cultures, but that's not who we are overall. Americans work hard, long hours; we're busy; and we don't generally have the time to behave like the French or any other culture.

Many public health professionals say our environment is responsible for our weight woes, believing that the abundance of fast-food restaurants, our addiction to eating out, and the proliferation of high-calorie convenience foods are all to blame.

This may all be true, but with *The Diet Detective's All-American Diet,* you'll learn how to flip the switch and use your environment to your *advantage.* We all know that eating out on a regular basis makes us vulnerable to weight gain because the food is often loaded with hidden calories, fat, and sugar, and the portions are excessively large. *The Diet Detective's All-American Diet* provides calorie-controlled options that are available at fast-food and casual dining establishments and shows you how to fit your favorite choices into your diet. On this diet, you can hit the snack, ready-to-eat, canned, and frozen food aisles at the grocery store, pick up fast food, dine out at your favorite restaurants, and eat your breakfast on the run. You just have to make the right choices. And this book will show you exactly how.

DIET DETECTIVE'S WHAT YOU NEED TO KNOW

EATING OUT

While there are foods from a variety of restaurants on the Build-a-Meal lists, restaurant foods are generally higher in calories, sodium, fat, and sugar than ready-to-eat items available at the grocery. Therefore, you will notice that most of the choices in the meal plans are not from restaurants. Try not to eat out more than three times per week. You can always take a frozen meal to work, keep it in the freezer, and microwave it. Or you can get a compact refrigerator with a small freezer to keep in your office for about $100 to $150.

This book is about using your cultural assets to your advantage and learning how to live, eat, and lose weight the American way. *The Diet Detective's All-American Diet* meal plans are made up of *regular* foods—not costly, hard-to-find specialty items. The Diet Detective's plan is easy to follow, often less expensive, certainly more accessible, and infinitely more practical than food-delivery programs or any other commercially available diet program.

The average American spends almost 9½ hours a day getting ready for bed and sleeping, 8 hours working (4 hours actually doing work), 2½ hours watching TV, 1 hour socializing, and only 1½ hours eating and drinking—not very much time, considering that eating is probably one of our most important activities. That means that most people don't have time for low-cal cooking. Rushing to get dinner on the table between work, soccer, ballet class, and bedtime is what often leads us to rely on takeout, fast food, and easy-to-fix convenience foods.

For years, I've been helping people simplify what they need to do to reach their weight-loss goals. Whether it's in my weekly column, the Diet Detective, which appears in more than 100 media outlets, or on my Web site, DietDetective.com (in partnership with Everdayhealth.com), I hunt out easy ways to avoid weight gain and calorie overload so you can continue to eat fast food, go to your favorite casual dining restaurants, eat takeout, have dessert—and still lose weight. I know you're tired and you want a simple formula that allows you to lose weight without radically altering your life—and that's exactly what the Diet Detective's Build-a-Meal Plan provides. All you have to do is figure out your calorie level by using the formula on page 10, choose a meal plan based on that, walk at least 30 minutes per day, and begin losing weight. Once you reach your goal weight, you will start the more flexible Build-a-Meal maintenance program.

The packaged entrées and restaurant foods among the Build-a-Meal options provide a reasonable alternative to eating out. The packaged foods' preparation requires only a few minutes in a microwave oven, and the portions are controlled. This means you can scarf down the entire meal without any guilt.

Not only that, but portion-controlled meals help you to recognize appropriate serving sizes. Once you're familiar with the size of a 300-calorie entrée, you'll have a better idea of how much you should be eating the next time you go out to dinner, or even when you're eating food you cooked at home. In fact, studies appearing in the journals *Obesity Research* and *Diabetes, Obesity and Metabolism* found that convenient prepackaged meals provided an uncomplicated weight-loss method for study participants.

DIET DETECTIVE'S WHAT YOU NEED TO KNOW

SEVERAL RESEARCH STUDIES SUPPORT THIS TYPE OF PROGRAM

You do not need to be a nutritionist, university professor, scientist, medical doctor, or diet guru to understand that if you eat portion-controlled meals created by the top food companies in the world, you will lose weight, but there are many scientific studies supporting this plan's efficacy.

- **"Use of packaged entrées as part of a weight-loss diet in overweight men: an 8-week randomized clinical trial"**
  "Our data suggest that the meal replacement diet plan evaluated was an effective strategy for producing robust initial weight loss and for achieving improvements in a number of health-related parameters during weight maintenance, including inflammation and oxidative stress, two key factors more recently shown to underlie our most common chronic diseases."

  —Diabetes, Obesity and Metabolism

- **"Use of portion-controlled entrées enhances weight loss in women"**
  "Consumption of portion-controlled entrées resulted in greater losses of weight and fat, thereby reducing cardiovascular disease risk. Accurate portion control is an important factor in weight-loss success, and use of packaged entrées is an effective method of achieving this."

  —Obesity Research

- **"Efficacy of meal replacements versus a standard food-based diet for weight loss in type 2 diabetes: a controlled clinical trial"**
  "A diet using portion-controlled meal replacements yielded significantly greater initial weight loss and less regain after 1 year of maintenance than a standard, self-selected, food-based diet."

  —The Diabetes Educator

- **"Do food provisions packaged in single-servings reduce energy intake at breakfast during a brief behavioral weight-loss intervention?"**
  Research shows that single-serving packages may help reduce energy intake at breakfast.
  —Journal of the American Dietetic Association

- **"Ready-to-eat cereal used as a meal replacement promotes weight loss in humans"**
  Research shows that easy, ready-to-eat cereals help you lose weight when consumed as a portion-controlled meal replacement.
  —Journal of the American College of Nutrition

Diet Detective's
All-American Diet Cheat Sheet

Here is a quick guide to everything you're going to need to do to make this diet work for you.

1. **Make a solid commitment to stick to the plan.** Mark the date you'll begin on your calendar (and don't make it a month from now!). Put your commitment down in writing and enlist the support of family and friends. Tell everyone about your goals and what you are doing so they can encourage you and help you stay on track if you start to stray.

2. **Start with your 21-Day Jump Start Program.** I know you really want to see results—and, in fact, being pleased with your initial results will help to boost your confidence in your ability to lose weight, which will contribute to your overall success. So, here's the key to jump-starting your diet. Women should use the 1,200-calorie Build-a-Meal plan, and men should stick to the 1,600-calorie Build-a-Meal plan. Abiding by these plans should result in the rapid weight loss that will help give you the confidence and motivation you need to continue!

   After this "initiation" period, you'll move on and figure out your daily calorie needs.

DIET DETECTIVE'S WHAT YOU NEED TO KNOW

CALORIES HAVE A BAD RAP

The word *calories* may conjure up images of all the sinful foods you shouldn't be eating. *The Diet Detective's All-American Diet* is here to help you appreciate calories rather than considering them the enemy. Calories should be thought of as energy that keeps you going. The only problem is that if you eat too many of them, you end up stockpiling unused energy, and that's what turns into fat.

3. **Put the Diet Detective's Build-a-Meal Plan into action.** Look at the lists beginning on page 64 and simply choose your breakfast entrée and side(s), a

DIET DETECTIVE'S WHAT YOU NEED TO KNOW

USE A RANGE, AND RELAX!

Keep in mind, your goal calorie level is a range. (For example, if you're on a 1,200-calorie plan, you can go up to 1,250 calories. Why? I don't think you need to match the calorie levels for each meal exactly. You will give up quickly if you feel like they need to conform to the specific parameters exactly. So you will notice that the sample plans are not exact. Just stay within a range from 1,200 to 1,250—and you're good to go!

midmorning snack, your lunch entrée and side(s), an afternoon snack, your dinner entrée and side(s), and a dessert, along with your beverages.

You will see that even though fruits and vegetables are generally considered side dishes, I have listed them in a separate category. That's because I want to make sure you include as many of them as possible in your meal plan. In selecting sides and snacks, always look at the fruits-and-vegetables list first (page 167). Fruits and vegetables are packed with fiber, which helps fill you up— exactly what you are looking for when you're trying to lose weight. For example, if your plan calls for a 100-calorie morning snack, try to choose one from the 100-calorie fruit and vegetable choices. Depending on your calorie allotment, you may even be able to have more than one serving of fruits and vegetables.

I also suggest you select only calorie-free beverages (club soda, unsweetened iced tea, water, etc.), but I have included lists of beverages with calories. Lastly, keep in mind that condiments have calories, too, and need to be taken into account when planning your meal—that's why they're listed as sides.

Are you interested in mostly vegetarian options? Low-carb foods? Sodium-controlled foods? Make sure to check for the symbols under the foods of your choice. All the Build-a-Meal plan foods are coded so that you can tailor your personal food plan accordingly.

    a.   Vegetarian =

    b.   Low Carb =

    c.   Sodium Controlled=

4. **Find your favorites.** Experiment and sample different foods. Some of the entrées or sides will not be to your liking—that's fine. Just do not overeat while

sampling—no sampling three or four meals at a time. Eventually you will find your favorites; stock up on those. You can even order them by the case if you want. For instance, Amazon.com offers Lean Cuisine, Healthy Choice, Amy's (soups), Weight Watchers Smart Ones, and many others. Ordering online means the foods will come directly to your door, which will make weight loss even easier.

5. **Create a weekly planning guide.** DO NOT SKIP THIS STEP! Take a look at the Weekly Planning Guide on page 27. Make sure you fill in every detail. Planning your meals in advance is extremely important because it leaves less room for things to go wrong—which is usually when people fall off the wagon.

6. **Create a weekly shopping list** (see page 28) This will ensure that all the foods on your weekly menu make it to your cupboard, fridge, and freezer. Go to the supermarket and stock up on your favorites.

7. **Weigh yourself.** Do this on the very first morning of your first day, before eating anything but after using the bathroom. Write down your starting weight. At the end of each week, record your weight. Try to be consistent about weighing in on the same day of the week at around the same time of day.

DIET DETECTIVE'S WHAT YOU NEED TO KNOW

LEARNING AND PLANNING MEALS INCREASES FOOD SATISFACTION

Having prior experience that a meal will be satisfying helps to ensure that it actually *is* satisfying, according to research from the University of Bristol, England. What this means is that when you plan your meals, it's a good idea to make sure you believe they will fill you up. My best advice is to experiment with different healthy meals to see which ones are most satisfying to *you*.

8. **Walk.** Yes, walk every single day for at least 30 minutes MORE than you were walking before you started the plan.

9. **Evaluate.** If you're not losing at least 1 pound per week, you need to reevaluate your meal plan and choose one that's 50 to 100 calories lower. *But under no circumstances should you eat fewer than 1,200 calories per day.* Not only is this

not considered healthy for most adults, but also it will cause your metabolism to slow down, which will make it harder to lose weight. Your body slows down your metabolism if it believes you are starving, and if you slash too many calories, that's exactly what will happen.

10. **Calculate your daily calorie needs for your Build-a-Meal menu plan.** When you are finished with the 21-Day Jump Start, it's time to calculate your calorie needs. This number is tailored to your body and your activity level, and it will help you get a good idea of where you need to be to move into the second phase of weight loss.

   a. Are you ACTIVE or NOT VERY ACTIVE?

   IF YOU ARE ACTIVE (i.e., you walk or do some form of exercise for at least 30 minutes each day):

   Multiply your weight x 15

   OR

   IF YOU ARE NOT VERY ACTIVE (i.e., you do NOT walk for at least 30 minutes every day):

   Multiply your weight x 12

   Do you want a more accurate calculation of calorie needs?
   Go to this Web site: www.goo.gl/cKKMg, then just follow the next steps!

   b. What number did you get? Write it here _____.

   c. Now, subtract 500.

   d. Write that number here _____.

This is the number of calories you will use for your Build-a-Meal plan to lose weight.

Example (Not Very Active):
You weigh 180.
Multiply 180 by 12 = 2,160
Now subtract 500 = 1,660

You are on a 1,600-calorie plan. (Round down to the nearest plan. *Never* eat fewer than 1,200 calories per day.)

Example (Active):
You weigh 180.
Multiply 180 by 15 = 2,700
Now subtract 500 = 2,200

You are on a 2,200-calorie plan. (Round down to the nearest plan. *Never* eat fewer than 1,200 calories per day.)

11. **Now lose weight and keep it off!** Eat the meals you choose and watch the weight drop off your body week after week. Once you reach your goal weight, move on to Phase 3—maintenance.

DIET DETECTIVE'S WHAT YOU NEED TO KNOW

THERE ARE NO MEAL PLANS FOR FEWER THAN 1,200 CALORIES OR MORE THAN 2,500 CALORIES

Never eat FEWER THAN 1,200 calories per day, even when you're on the 21-Day Jump Start program.

If your plan ADDS UP to more than 2,500 calories per day (the highest number I recommend), you should check with your physician about the appropriate calorie level for you to lose weight.

You should always check with your physician before starting this or any weight-loss program.

Move and Burn

Research shows that a combination of healthier food choices and physical activity (mostly walking) is what helps people lose weight and keep it off. In addition, an increase in physical activity offers other benefits, including cardiovascular health, and strength training can add muscle, which can burn extra calories at rest. (Each pound of muscle added will increase the calories your body burns by about 30 to 50 calories per day.)

Walk It Off

After decades of being told that "exercise" requires a serious commitment of time and sweat (and sometimes aches, pains, and tears), you may find it difficult to believe that something as simple as going for a walk could improve your health and help you lose weight.

I must admit, I never thought much of walking. I mean, it was always a necessary means to an end if I had to get from Point A to Point B, but as a form of exercise, it seemed a bit weak.

Nevertheless, research has shown that walking works. A study published in the *American Journal of Public Health* found that people who live in the suburbs—and therefore drive everywhere—weigh on average 6.3 pounds more than urbanites who are able to walk more. In fact, Manhattan, the heart of New York City, has one of the lowest obesity rates in the country, and many experts attribute this to the fact that so many of its residents walk regularly.

There is nothing like going for a nice walk. You can do it anywhere. And you can accomplish other tasks at the same time, such as shopping, picking up your cleaning, or stopping for a quart of low-fat milk. "Walking is a flexible and available exercise that's easy to incorporate into your everyday life. And there are additional benefits. For instance, your body will preferentially lose more fat and hang on to more muscle when you start a walking program (or any exercise program)," says Ross E. Andersen, PhD, a professor of geriatric medicine at Johns Hopkins University School of Medicine.

Additionally, walking helps you become more mindful of what you're eating so you can manage your weight better. "When you consciously increase your physical activity, you become more aware of your surroundings, and you're less likely to grab that candy bar at the checkout counter," says Dr. Andersen. And, he goes on to explain, it also seems to be the "gateway" to more vigorous exercise, which leads to even greater overall results. "Self-confidence increases after you start a walking program, and as your self-confidence increases, you start including more fitness in your life."

And get this—you burn only about 20 percent more calories when you run a mile than you do when you walk a mile. So walking means less sweat and less muscle stress at about the same calorie expenditure. Not bad, right?

In fact, recent studies have highlighted the many benefits of going out for a stroll. Walking has fewer risks of injury than fast-paced jogging; walkers get a better overall workout than most runners; and age does not serve as an impediment—both young and old can participate and reap the rewards.

In a key study published in the *Journal of the American Medical Association,* Dr. Andersen showed that a program of diet plus lifestyle activity can be a suitable alternative and offer health benefits similar to diet plus vigorous activity for overweight individuals.

You might also want to consider another study from the University of Pittsburgh, which found that easy physical activity burns calories and encourages weight loss just as effectively as high-intensity exercise. This means that slow walkers can burn calories despite their slower pace; it will just take them longer than brisk walkers to lose the same amount of weight.

"It appears that intensity is not the main factor impacting long-term weight loss or weight control. The more you walk, the better off you are in terms of losing weight," says John M. Jakicic, PhD, a professor at the School of Education at the University of Pittsburgh and author of the study. However, in order to lose weight, "you need to walk an additional 250 to 300 minutes per week over a period of four to five days," he cautions.

Not convinced yet? There was also a Duke University study that showed that you can walk for 30 minutes a day, not diet, and maintain your weight loss. And according to the National Weight Control Registry, which keeps an ongoing record of individuals who have managed to maintain weight loss for 5 years or more, a staggering 77 percent of successful losers use walking as their means of physical activity. Let's face it—running for 30 minutes straight isn't something most of us would look forward to doing on a regular basis.

Be Creative

Malls, parks, paths, trails, and even your very own neighborhood's sidewalks are perfect sites for a 10-minute, 15-minute, or even 30-minute walk. On rainy days, malls can be converted into indoor tracks. Walk the entire mall for a good 30 minutes at moderate speed. The level flooring (meaning fewer injuries) and climate-controlled environment are excellent motivators for using the mall as a walking spot.

Make It Scenic

If walking around the mall isn't your thing, try locating walking tours around your city. Sightseeing is very distracting, and before you know it, you'll have walked a few miles while discovering more about your neighborhood or even a new neighborhood.

Research also shows that the more scenic your walks are, the more you'll want to take them. Seek out the best-looking walking routes. Some parks offer trails specifically designed for hikers. Grass and dirt paths are flat and reduce shock and stress on your feet. If you want a little extra challenge, find paths with hills, take a few breaks, and walk for an hour instead of just 30 minutes.

Make It Social

Various communities sponsor walking clubs; take advantage of those resources and join. Walking in a group will increase motivation and distraction and will help you challenge yourself by keeping up with the others.

Make It Practical

A common complaint is being too busy to exercise. So fit in your walking with things you need to do anyway. The dog has to get out, so why not take him for a walk? The kids need to go to school—why not walk them to the bus stop? If it's too far to walk all the way to the store or wherever you need to go, drive or take the bus halfway and walk the remaining distance.

Get Good Walking Shoes

Before you go outside and start counting your steps, keep in mind that you need to have the proper shoes. Podiatrists suggest getting cross-trainers or specific walking or running shoes. Stay away from those "designer" shoes that are all looks but no support.

DIET DETECTIVE'S WHAT YOU NEED TO KNOW

CALORIE BURNING PER MINUTE OF EXERCISE

	EASY	MODERATE	BRISK/FAST
Walking:	4 cal/min	4.5 cal/min	5 cal/min
Biking:	7 cal/min	11 cal/min	13.5 cal/min
Running:	9 cal/min	13 cal/min	15 cal/min

If you're already doing these things, that's wonderful, but remember, that doesn't count as an increase in physical activity. You have to *add new activities* to increase your caloric expenditure.

Overcome Environmental Barriers

It's important to understand your environmental constraints and barriers. The biggest barriers or excuses for not walking, according to a study in the *Journal of the American College of Sports Medicine,* are the lack of walking trails or sidewalks, not seeing other people exercising, unattended dogs, and heavy traffic. "Learn how to work around these obstacles by setting goals and researching your area," says Ross C. Brownson, PhD, professor of epidemiology at St. Louis University School of Public Health in Missouri and a coauthor of the study.

Ask yourself the following questions about where you live:

- Does my neighborhood have public or private recreation facilities (such as parks with walking or hiking trails)? Are they in good condition? Can I see myself using them?
- Does my local public school have any facilities I can use (such as a track)?
- Does my neighborhood shopping mall have walking programs available?
- Do concerns about safety at the public recreation facilities in my community influence my not using them? Do I have safety concerns about walking in my neighborhood? What could I do to overcome these safety issues?
- Do the parks near my home have walking or hiking trails? Bike paths?

To locate hiking and/or biking trails in your area, log on to www.traillink.com.

Exercises You Can Do at Home Right Now

In addition to walking every day, you need to do strength training to get the best results. A convenient at-home exercise program you can stick to three times a week is certainly better than going to the gym once a month. Here are several suggested exercises you should try to weave into your everyday life. Some of these exercises require resistance bands or tubes—when using these bands, make sure to keep the tension the same throughout the entire range of motion. Depending on the band, tension can increase toward the end of the exercise.

Make sure you consult a physician before starting any exercise program. Whenever you engage in any kind of exercise, you should feel the intended muscles being activated. You should not feel lower-back pain or pain in any area the exercise is not intended to affect. Finally, always be in control, and don't do extra repetitions of any exercise when that would mean not maintaining perfect form.

Plank and Side Plank

Targets: Abdominals, scapular stabilizers, back extensors

Equipment: None

Starting position: Begin on your hands and knees with your hands a little more than shoulder-width apart and slightly in front of your shoulders.

Movement: Extend one leg at a time, coming to balance on the balls of your feet, as in the "up" part of a pushup. Contract your abdominals so that your back is parallel to the floor. Keep your head and neck in line with your spine.

Side plank: From the plank position, bring your feet together so that they are touching one another and roll onto the outside of your right foot while lifting your left arm up toward the ceiling. Repeat on the other side.

How many: Start by holding for 15 seconds, building up to 60 seconds, and do 1 repetition.

Cat Camel

Targets: Spinal mobility, mid- to lower back, hips

Equipment: None

Starting position: Start on your hands and knees. Make sure your knees are directly under your hips and your hands are directly under your shoulders.

Movement: Inhale and look up as you let your stomach soften toward the floor while arching your back and letting your buttocks lift toward the ceiling as if forming the letter U. Then, as you exhale, let your head and buttocks round toward the floor so that your spine humps and your stomach is concave. Repeat inhaling and exhaling with slow, controlled movements.

How many: 2 sets of 10 repetitions

Pushup

Targets: Pectoralis major, front deltoids, triceps, chest, abdominals

Equipment: None

Starting position: Begin facedown with your weight on your hands and the balls of your feet. Place your hands a little wider than shoulder-width apart and slightly in front of your shoulders, and keep your legs together. Contract your abdominals so your back is parallel to the floor. Keep your head and neck in line with your spine.

Movement: Inhale as you lower your chest as close to the floor as possible. Exhale as you squeeze your chest muscles inward to return to the starting position.

How many: 3 sets of 10 repetitions

Squat

Targets: Buttocks, hamstrings, quadriceps, legs

Equipment: None, or you can use dumbbells.

Starting position: Stand with your feet a little wider than shoulder-width apart and your arms hanging at your sides. Keep your torso erect and your body weight over your heels.

Movement: Inhale as you bend your knees and lower your body as if to sit in a chair until your thighs are as close to parallel to the floor as possible. Do not go lower than this, or you will put too much stress on your knees. Exhale as you squeeze your buttocks and come back to the starting position. Always keep your knees in line with your second toe. (I realize that "your second toe" may sound strange, but if your knees extended to your big toe, it would be too far.) Do not let your knees extend over your toes. Variation: Hold dumbbells in your hands.

How many: 2 sets of 10 repetitions

Ball Leg Raise

Targets: Abductors, buttocks, torso, core
Equipment: Exercise/stability ball (25 centimeters)
Starting position: Lie faceup on the floor. Hold an exercise ball between your knees, keeping your knees above your hips and your arms at your sides, palms facing up.

Movement: Exhale as you lift your hips and pull your knees toward your chin with the ball between your legs. Make sure to concentrate on using your abdominal muscles to bring the ball toward your chin. Inhale as you slowly lower to the starting position.

How many: 2 sets of 10 repetitions

Scissors or Flutter Kick

Targets: Torso, core (including abdominals)
Equipment: None
Starting position: Lie faceup on the floor with your hands at your sides, palms down. Pull your abdominals in so you can lengthen your back.

Movement: Lift your legs about 3 inches off the floor. Exhale as you rapidly move your legs up and down (moving your right and left legs in opposite directions) in a scissorlike motion between 3 and 6 inches. Inhale as you slowly return to the starting position.

How many: 2 sets of 10 repetitions

Pelvic Tilt/Hip Extension/Bridge

Targets: Lower body, buttocks, hamstrings, adductors (stabilize hip joints)

Equipment: None

Starting position: Lie on your back with your knees bent and your feet on the floor. Make sure your feet are in line with your hips and your toes are pointing forward.

Movement: Keeping your feet flat and pressing all four corners firmly into the floor, lift your hips up off the floor. Exhale as you squeeze your buttocks and tighten your lower abdominal muscles to lift your pelvis off the floor. Inhale as you lower your pelvis and return to the starting position. Make sure to use your glute muscles (buttocks) to lift your hips.

How many: 2 sets of 10 repetitions

Shoulder Press

Targets: Shoulders, including the anterior, medial, and posterior deltoids, and triceps

Equipment: Resistance bands, tubes, or dumbbells and a stability ball

Starting position: Sit on a stability ball (or a chair) with your feet slightly wider than shoulder-width apart. Center a resistance band or tube beneath both feet, or you can use 5- to 10-pound dumbbells. Grasp the handles and bring your hands level with your ears, elbows bent 90 degrees and out to the sides: You're sort of making a W with your arms. Contract your abdominals and maintain an erect posture. Make sure to keep your head and back straight.

Movement: Exhale as you raise your hands out and up over your head. Tighten your abdominals as you press your arms toward the ceiling until only a slight bend remains in your elbows. Do not touch your hands together at the top of the move. Inhale as you slowly return to the starting position.

How many: 1 set of 10 repetitions

Lateral Raise

Targets: Shoulders, including anterior, medial, and posterior deltoids

Equipment: Resistance bands, tubes, or dumbbells

Starting position: While standing with feet shoulder-width apart, center the resistance band or tube beneath both feet (or grab the dumbbells). Keep your knees soft and slightly bent. Grasp the handles and bring your hands to your sides with your arms hanging straight down and your palms facing in toward your sides. Keep your chest up and shoulders back and upright.

Movement: Inhale, then exhale and move your arms out from your sides (keeping arms straight) until your hands are at shoulder level. You're bringing your arms out to your sides until they are parallel to the floor, so that you are forming a letter T. Lower your arms back down to the sides of your legs and repeat. Make sure to tighten your trunk by contracting your core muscles (midsection), and keep your back straight.

How many: 2 sets of 10 repetitions

Biceps Curl

Targets: Biceps

Equipment: Resistance bands, tubes, or dumbbells

Starting position: Stand with your feet shoulder-width apart, knees comfortable, pelvis tucked, shoulders dropped, and chin level. Center the resistance band/tube under both feet and grasp the handles (or dumbbells) with your palms facing forward and your arms extended straight down from your shoulders. Keep your elbows anchored to your sides.

Movement: Inhale, then exhale as you bend your elbows, palms facing up, to bring your hands three-fourths of the way to your shoulders. Inhale as you return to the starting position.

How many: 2 sets of 10 repetitions

Pullup

Targets: Back muscles, including latissimus dorsi, teres major, middle trapezius, and rhomboids

Equipment: Pullup bar

Starting position: First of all, be careful grasping the bar—you might want to step on a bench. (If you use a stool or bench, bend your knees so it's out of the way after you grasp the bar.) Grasp the bar with a firm grip, hands slightly wider than shoulder-width apart. If your legs do not clear the floor in the dead-hang starting position, bend your knees to raise your feet. Cross your ankles for added stability.

Movement: Exhale as you raise your body in a single, smooth motion by pulling the bar toward your chest until your chin is above the bar. Do not bicycle (lift your feet alternately) or kick your legs while lifting your body. Inhale as you slowly return to the starting position.

How many: Try to do as many as you can with good form, without swinging your body. The goal is to do 3 sets of 5 repetitions.

Forward Lunge

Targets: Buttocks, hamstrings, quadriceps, abductors

Equipment: None

Starting position: Stand with feet together, hands on hips.

Movement: Inhale as you step forward with your right leg and bend your right knee at a 90-degree angle. Don't lean back before stepping forward, and keep your trunk in front of your hips when you do move forward. Keep your knee directly above your toes during the downward movement to avoid overstressing the knee joint. Exhale as you push off your toes to return to the starting position. Keep an upright posture throughout the exercise. Make sure that your head, shoulders, hips, and ankles are all aligned. Then repeat with your left leg forward.

How many: 2 sets of 10 repetitions on each side

Build-a-Meal

Build-a-Meal
Eating Program
with Sample Meal Plans

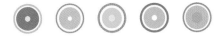

Once you've used the formula on page 10 to determine how many calories you should be eating each day, look at the lists starting on page 64 showing your meal and snack choices. Now select an appropriate week's worth of breakfast, lunch, dinner, and snack items from those lists. On pages 30 through 61, I've provided sample meal plans for each plan level to show you how this works. Do not think that you can wing it each day.

I know you think you can carry this book with you and simply choose your lunch entrée at lunch time—but it will *not* work. You need to plan your entire week's worth of eating ahead of time. Can you change your mind? Of course. But it's important to have the plan in place. So make it easy on yourself by taking 30 minutes or so to sit down and figure your entire week's worth of eating. The Build-a-Meal lists make it easy to do this, but if you don't do it, you will end up scrambling to find food when you're hungry—the worst possible time if you're trying to diet.

The same holds true for exercise. If you don't chart your exercise plan in advance, you probably won't do it. So the Weekly Planning Guide also includes a place to write down what you're going to do each day.

DIET DETECTIVE'S WHAT YOU NEED TO KNOW

EXCHANGES

If, for example, your plan says you can have a 100-calorie snack, feel free to choose two 50-calorie sides instead. You can also do this with all the snack choices. One note of caution: Make sure you don't start a calorie slide by adding an extra 25 calories here and there. Keep to the total number of calories on your plan.

WEEKLY PLANNING GUIDE							
MEALS	MON	TUES	WED	THURS	FRI	SAT	SUN
BREAKFAST							
Breakfast Entrée							
Breakfast Side Try to include a fruit or vegetable as your side, if you can.							
No-Calorie Drink (Just because you can have a caloric drink does not mean you have to have one—save the calories.)							
MORNING SNACK							
Try to include a fruit or vegetable in your snack.							
LUNCH							
Lunch Entrée							
Lunch Side(s) (Try to have soup or salad.)							
No-Calorie Drink (Just because you can have a caloric drink does not mean you have to have one—save the calories.)							
AFTERNOON SNACK							
Try to include a fruit or vegetable in your snack							
DINNER							
Dinner Entrée							
Dinner Side(s) (Try to have soup or salad)							
No-Calorie Drink (Just because you can have a caloric drink does not mean you have to have one—save the calories.))							
DESSERT							
(Only if it's on your plan or if you exchange for a side.)							
TOTAL CALORIES							
Prep for Next Day's Meals What you have to prepare or pack for the next day's meals							
Walking or Other Extra Activity							
Minutes							
Weight							

WEEKLY SHOPPING LIST

Entrées	Sides	Snacks	Desserts	Beverages

ALL-AMERICAN DIET

How to Create
Your Own
Build-a-Meal Plan

1,200-CALORIE MEAL PLAN

	CALORIES
BREAKFAST	
Breakfast Entrée	250
Drink	25
Total Breakfast calories	**275**
MORNING SNACK	
Total Snack calories	**50**
LUNCH	
Lunch Entrée	300
Drink	0
Total Lunch calories	**300**
AFTERNOON SNACK	
Total Snack calories	**50**
DINNER	
Fruit or Vegetable	50
Dinner Entrée	350
Dinner Side(s)	50
Drink	25
Total Dinner calories	**475**
DESSERT	
Total Dessert calories	**50**
TOTAL	**1,200**

SAMPLE 1,200-CALORIE MEAL PLAN	CALORIES
BREAKFAST	
Entrée: Dunkin' Donuts Sausage, Egg White and Cheese Wake-Up Wrap	240
Drink: Dunkin' Donuts Iced Coffee (Medium)	20
MORNING SNACK	
Snack: Mott's No Sugar Added Natural Apple Sauce	50
Drink: Water	0
LUNCH	
Entrée: Subway Roasted Chicken Noodle Soup	310
Drink: Diet Pepsi	0
AFTERNOON SNACK	
Snack: Ready Pac Carrots with Ranch Dip Snack Pac	70
Drink: Water	0
DINNER	
Vegetable: Fresh Express 5-Lettuce Mix (1 bag)	45
Side: Wish-Bone Salad Spritzers Balsamic Breeze Vinaigrette Dressing (10 sprays)	10
Entrée: Amy's Roasted Vegetable Lasagna	350
Side: Campbell's Vegetable Beef Soup at Hand	70
DESSERT	
Dessert: Popsicle Ice Pops Jolly Rancher (1 pop)	45
Drink: Water	0
TOTAL:	**1,210**

1,300-CALORIE MEAL PLAN	
	CALORIES
BREAKFAST	
Breakfast Entrée	250
Breakfast Side(s)	50
Drink	25
Total Breakfast calories	325
MORNING SNACK	
Total Snack calories	50
LUNCH	
Lunch Entrée	300
Lunch Side(s)	50
Drink	0
Total Lunch calories	350
AFTERNOON SNACK	
Total Snack calories	50
DINNER	
Fruit or Vegetable	50
Dinner Entrée	350
Dinner Side(s)	50
Drink	25
Total Dinner calories	475
DESSERT	
Total Dessert calories	50
TOTAL	1,300

SAMPLE 1,300-CALORIE MEAL PLAN	CALORIES
BREAKFAST	
Entrée: ½ cup Post Grape-Nuts Cereal with ½ cup skim milk	240
Side: Oscar Mayer Fully Cooked Bacon (4 slices)	70
Fruit: 50 blueberries	39
Drink: Starbucks 16-Ounce Black Coffee	5
MORNING SNACK	
Fruit: Orange	69
Drink: Water (Reminder: Drink more water.)	0
LUNCH	
Entrée: McDonald's Grilled Chicken Chipotle BBQ Snack Wrap	260
Side: McDonald's Side Salad with Newman's Own Southwest Dressing	55
Drink: Water	0
AFTERNOON SNACK	
Snack: Campbell's Chicken & Stars Soup at Hand	70
Drink: Water	0
DINNER	
Vegetable: Fresh Express Baby Spinach (1 bag)	40
Side: Wish-Bone Salad Spritzers Balsamic Breeze Vinaigrette Dressing (10 sprays)	10
Entrée: Lean Cuisine Casual Cuisine Four Cheese Pizza	350
Side: Green Giant Just for One Broccoli & Cheese	40
DESSERT	
Dessert: Popsicle Flavored Juice Ice Pops Scribblers, Assorted Flavors (2 pops)	60
Drink: Water	0
TOTAL	**1,308**

1,350-CALORIE MEAL PLAN	
	CALORIES
BREAKFAST	
Breakfast Entrée	250
Breakfast Side(s)	50
Drink	25
Total Breakfast calories	**225**
MORNING SNACK	
Total Snack calories	**50**
LUNCH	
Lunch Entrée	300
Lunch Side(s)	50
Drink	0
Total Lunch calories	**350**
AFTERNOON SNACK	
Total Snack calories	**50**
DINNER	
Fruit or Vegetable	50
Dinner Entrée	350
Dinner Side(s)	50
Drink	25
Total Dinner calories	**475**
DESSERT	
Total Dessert calories	**100**
TOTAL	**1,350**

SAMPLE 1,350-CALORIE MEAL PLAN	CALORIES
BREAKFAST	
Entrée: Aunt Jemima Pancakes Made with Whole Grain (3 pancakes)	240
Side: Stonyfield Farm YoKids Lowfat Strawberry Squeezer	50
Drink: Starbucks Grande Black Coffee	5
MORNING SNACK	
Fruit: Sunsweet 60 Calorie Packs Prunes (1 pouch)	60
Drink: Water	0
LUNCH	
Entrée: Taco Bell Beef Enchirito	360
Drink: Water	0
AFTERNOON SNACK	
Snack: Kraft Polly-O String Cheese, Mozzarella	70
Drink: Water	0
DINNER	
Vegetable: Cascadian Farm Whole Petite Green Beans (1 box)	68
Entrée: Healthy Choice Café Steamers Sweet Sesame Chicken	340
Side: Amy's Low Fat Vegetable Barley Soup (½ can)	70
Drink: Water	0
DESSERT:	
Dessert: Dreyer's Tangerine Fruit Bar	80
TOTAL	**1,343**

1,400-CALORIE MEAL PLAN

	CALORIES
BREAKFAST	
Breakfast Entrée	250
Breakfast Side(s)	50
Drink	25
Total Breakfast calories	**325**
MORNING SNACK	
Total Snack calories	**50**
LUNCH	
Lunch Entrée	350
Lunch Side(s)	50
Drink	0
Total Lunch calories	**400**
AFTERNOON SNACK	
Total Snack calories	**50**
DINNER	
Fruit or Vegetable	50
Dinner Entrée	350
Dinner Side(s)	50
Drink	25
Total Dinner calories	**475**
DESSERT	
Total Dessert calories	**100**
TOTAL	**1,400**

SAMPLE
1,400-CALORIE MEAL PLAN

	CALORIES
BREAKFAST	
Entrée: Amy's Breakfast Burrito	270
Side: Dole Tropical Fruit Cup	60
Drink: Starbucks Grande Black Coffee	5
MORNING SNACK	
Fruit: 20 red or green grapes	66
Drink: Water	0
LUNCH	
Entrée: Healthy Choice Fresh Mixers Rotini and Zesty Marinara Sauce	300
Side: Amy's Fat Free Chunky Vegetable Soup (½ can)	60
Drink: Water	0
AFTERNOON SNACK	
Snack: Ready Pac Carrots with Ranch Dip Snack Pac	70
Drink: Water	0
DINNER	
Vegetable: Birds Eye Steamfresh Singles Super Sweet Corn (1 bag)	80
Entrée: Campbell's Creamy Chicken & Dumplings Chunky Soup Microwaveable Bowl	380
Side: Medium tomato	22
Drink: Water	0
DESSERT:	
Dessert: Skinny Cow French Vanilla Truffle Low Fat Ice Cream Bar	100
TOTAL	**1,413**

BUILD-A-MEAL

1,450-CALORIE MEAL PLAN	
	CALORIES
BREAKFAST	
Breakfast Entrée	300
Breakfast Side(s)	50
Drink	25
Total Breakfast calories	**375**
MORNING SNACK	
Total Snack calories	**50**
LUNCH	
Lunch Entrée	350
Lunch Side(s)	50
Drink	0
Total Lunch calories	**400**
AFTERNOON SNACK	
Total Snack calories	**50**
DINNER	
Fruit or Vegetable	50
Dinner Entrée	350
Dinner Side(s)	50
Drink	25
Total Dinner calories	**475**
DESSERT	
Total Dessert calories	**100**
TOTAL	**1,450**

SAMPLE 1,450-CALORIE MEAL PLAN	CALORIES
BREAKFAST	
Entrée: Lean Pockets Breakfast Sausage Egg & Cheese (1 piece)	280
Side: Del Monte Pineapple Tidbits Cup	70
Drink: Black coffee (12 ounces.)	5
MORNING SNACK	
Fruit: 1 cup blackberries	62
Drink: Water	0
LUNCH	
Entrée: Lean Cuisine Casual Cuisine Chicken Club Panini	360
Side: Campbell's Chicken & Stars Soup at Hand	70
Drink: Water	0
AFTERNOON SNACK	
Snack: Mott's Sliced Apples (1 bag)	57
Drink: Water	0
DINNER	
Vegetable: Del Monte Mixed Vegetables	70
Entrée: McDonald's Filet-O-Fish	380
Side: McDonald's Side Salad with Newman's Own Southwest Dressing	55
Drink: Water	0
DESSERT	
Dessert: Popsicle Flavored Ice Pops, Orange, Cherry, or Grape Flavored (1 pop)	45
TOTAL	**1,454**

1,500-CALORIE MEAL PLAN

	CALORIES
BREAKFAST	
Breakfast Entrée	300
Breakfast Side(s)	50
Drink	25
Total Breakfast calories	**375**
MORNING SNACK	
Morning Snack	50
Drink	25
Total Snack calories	**75**
LUNCH	
Lunch Entrée	350
Lunch Side(s)	50
Drink	25
Total Lunch calories	**425**
AFTERNOON SNACK	
Total Snack calories	**50**
DINNER	
Fruit or Vegetable	50
Dinner Entrée	350
Dinner Side(s)	50
Drink	25
Total Dinner calories	**475**
DESSERT	
Total Dessert calories	**100**
TOTAL	**1,500**

ALL-AMERICAN DIET

SAMPLE
1,500-CALORIE MEAL PLAN

	CALORIES
BREAKFAST	
Entrée: McDonald's Hotcakes	350
Side: Mott's Plus Antioxidants Pomegranate Apple Sauce	50
Drink: Black coffee (12 ounces)	5
MORNING SNACK	
Fruit: ½ red or white grapefruit	37
Drink: Water	0
LUNCH	
Entrée: Denny's Grilled Shrimp Skewers (4 skewers)	360
Fruit: Kiwi	52
Drink: Water	0
AFTERNOON SNACK	
Snack: Dole Cherry Mixed Fruit	70
Drink: Water	0
DINNER	
Vegetable: Green Giant Broccoli Florettes (1 package)	88
Entrée: Amy's Whole Meals Chili & Cornbread	340
Side: Campbell's Vegetable Beef Soup at Hand	70
Drink: Water	0
DESSERT:	
Dessert: Snack Pack Fat Free Tapioca	80
TOTAL	**1,502**

1,600-CALORIE MEAL PLAN	
	CALORIES
BREAKFAST	
Breakfast Entrée	300
Breakfast Side(s)	50
Drink	25
Total Breakfast calories	375
MORNING SNACK	
Morning Snack	50
Drink	25
Total Snack calories	75
LUNCH	
Lunch Entrée	350
Lunch Side(s)	50
Drink	25
Total Lunch calories	425
AFTERNOON SNACK	
Total Snack calories	100
DINNER	
Fruit or Vegetable	50
Dinner Entrée	400
Dinner Side(s)	50
Drink	25
Total Dinner calories	525
DESSERT	
Total Dessert calories	100
TOTAL	1,600

SAMPLE 1,600-CALORIE MEAL PLAN	CALORIES
BREAKFAST	
Entrée: Thomas' Blueberry Bagel	270
Side: I Can't Believe It's Not Butter! Spray	0
Side: ½ white or red grapefruit	37
Drink: Starbucks Grande Black Coffee	5
MORNING SNACK	
Fruit: 8 large strawberries	48
Drink: Water	0
LUNCH	
Entrée: Quiznos Veggie Sammie	340
Side: Quiznos Chicken Noodle Soup	110
Drink: Water	0
AFTERNOON SNACK	
Fruit: Banana	105
Drink: Water	0
DINNER	
Vegetable: Fresh Express Baby Spinach (1 package)	40
Vegetable: Medium green pepper	24
Vegetable: Medium tomato	22
Entrée: Healthy Choice Complete Meals Sweet & Sour Chicken	420
Side: Amy's Low Fat Vegetable Barley Soup (½ can)	70
Drink: Water	0
DESSERT	
Dessert: Weight Watchers English Toffee Crunch Ice Cream Bar	100
TOTAL	**1,591**

BUILD-A-MEAL

1,700-CALORIE MEAL PLAN	
	CALORIES
BREAKFAST	
Breakfast Entrée	300
Breakfast Side(s)	50
Drink	25
Total Breakfast calories	375
MORNING SNACK	
Morning Snack	100
Drink	25
Total Snack calories	125
LUNCH	
Lunch Entrée	350
Lunch Side(s)	50
Drink	25
Total Lunch calories	425
AFTERNOON SNACK	
Total Snack calories	100
DINNER	
Fruit or Vegetable	50
Dinner Entrée	400
Dinner Side(s)	100
Drink	25
Total Dinner calories	575
DESSERT	
Total Dessert calories	100
TOTAL	1,700

ALL-AMERICAN DIET

SAMPLE 1,700-CALORIE MEAL PLAN	CALORIES
BREAKFAST	
Entrée: McDonald's Egg, Ham & Cheese McMuffin	300
Side: Earth's Best Organic Yogurt Rice Crisp Cereal Bar, Banana	70
Side: Sunsweet 70 Calorie Packs Dried Apricots	70
Drink: Water	0
MORNING SNACK	
Snack: Ready Pac Ready Snax Apples, Granola & Yogurt Snack Pac	110
Drink: Water	0
LUNCH	
Entrée: KFC Extra Crispy Thigh	340
Side: Amy's Fat Free Chunky Vegetable Soup (½ can)	60
Drink: Water	0
AFTERNOON SNACK	
Fruit: Banana	105
Drink: Water	0
DINNER	
Vegetable: Taylor Organic Baby Spring Mix (1 bag)	40
Side: Wish-Bone Ranch Vinaigrette Dressing (10 sprays)	15
Side: Dole Sugar Snap Peas (½ package)	70
Entrée: Amy's Single Serve Cheese Pizza	420
Drink: Water	0
DESSERT	
Dessert: The Skinny Cow Caramel Truffle Ice Cream Bar	100
TOTAL	**1,705**

BUILD-A-MEAL

1,800-CALORIE MEAL PLAN	
	CALORIES
BREAKFAST	
Breakfast Entrée	300
Breakfast Side(s)	50
Drink	25
Total Breakfast calories	375
MORNING SNACK	
Morning Snack	100
Drink	25
Total Snack calories	125
LUNCH	
Lunch Entrée	350
Lunch Side(s)	50
Drink	25
Total Lunch calories	425
AFTERNOON SNACK	
Total Snack calories	150
DINNER	
Fruit or Vegetable	100
Dinner Entrée	400
Dinner Side(s)	100
Drink	25
Total Dinner calories	625
DESSERT	
Total Dessert calories	100
TOTAL	1,800

SAMPLE
1,800-CALORIE MEAL PLAN

	CALORIES
BREAKFAST	
Entrée: Jimmy Dean Bacon, Egg & Cheese Biscuit Sandwich	320
Side: Mott's Healthy Harvest No Sugar Added Peach Medley Apple Sauce	50
Drink: Water	0
MORNING SNACK	
Snack: Ready Pac Ready Snax Apples, Granola & Yogurt Snack Pac	100
Drink: Water	0
LUNCH	
Entrée: Rally's/Checkers Chili Cheese Dog	380
Side: Mott's Sliced Apples (1 bag)	57
Drink: Water	0
AFTERNOON SNACK	
Snack: Dole Fruit Crisps, Pineapple Mango (1 container)	150
Drink: Water	0
DINNER	
Vegetable: Birds Eye Steamfresh Broccoli Cuts (1 bag)	120
Entrée: Banquet Turkey Pot Pie	380
Side: Green Giant Just for One Peas and Corn in Basil Butter Sauce	80
Drink: Water	0
DESSERT	
Dessert: Weight Watchers Mint Chocolate Chip Ice Cream Cup	140
TOTAL	**1,777**

1,900-CALORIE MEAL PLAN

	CALORIES
BREAKFAST	
Breakfast Entrée	300
Breakfast Side(s)	50
Drink	25
Total Breakfast calories	**375**
MORNING SNACK	
Morning Snack	100
Drink	25
Total Snack calories	**125**
LUNCH	
Lunch Entrée	350
Lunch Side(s)	100
Drink	25
Total Lunch calories	**475**
AFTERNOON SNACK	
Total Snack calories	**150**
DINNER	
Fruit or Vegetable	100
Dinner Entrée	400
Dinner Side(s)	100
Drink	25
Total Dinner calories	**625**
DESSERT	
Total Dessert calories	**150**
TOTAL	**1,900**

SAMPLE 1,900-CALORIE MEAL PLAN	CALORIES
BREAKFAST	
Entrée: Jamba Juice 30-ounce Strawberry Nirvana Light Smoothie	300
Side: Earth's Best Organic Yogurt Rice Crisp Bars, Banana	70
Side: 20 grapes	66
MORNING SNACK	
Snack: Ocean Spray 100 Calorie Packs Craisins	100
Drink: Water	0
LUNCH	
Entrée: Progresso Traditional New England Clam Chowder (1 can)	360
Side: Emerald 100 Calorie Packs Natural Walnuts and Almonds (1 pouch)	100
Drink: Water	0
AFTERNOON SNACK	
Snack: Dole Fruit Crisps, Pineapple Mango (1 container)	150
Drink: Water	0
DINNER	
Entrée: Chili's Classic Sirloin	400
Side: Chili's Side of Broccoli	30
Side: Chili's Spicy Garlic and Lime, 6 pieces	150
Fruit: 8 strawberries	48
Drink: Water	0
DESSERT	
Dessert: Skinny Cow Mint with Fudge Low Fat Ice Cream Cone	150
TOTAL	**1,924**

2,000-CALORIE MEAL PLAN	
	CALORIES
BREAKFAST	
Breakfast Entrée	300
Breakfast Side(s)	50
Drink	25
Total Breakfast calories	**375**
MORNING SNACK	
Morning Snack	150
Drink	25
Total Snack calories	**175**
LUNCH	
Lunch Entrée	350
Lunch Side(s)	100
Lunch Drink	25
Total Lunch calories	**475**
AFTERNOON SNACK	
Total Snack calories	**150**
DINNER	
Fruit or Vegetable	100
Dinner Entrée	450
Dinner Side(s)	100
Dinner Drink	25
Total Dinner calories	**675**
DESSERT	
Total Dessert calories	**150**
TOTAL	**2,000**

SAMPLE 2,000-CALORIE MEAL PLAN	CALORIES
BREAKFAST	
Entrée: Dunkin' Donuts Grilled Cheese Flatbread Sandwich	380
Drink: Dunkin' Donuts Large Iced (16 ounces) Coffee	20
MORNING SNACK	
Snack: Yoplait Original Strawberry Banana Yogurt	170
Drink: Water	0
LUNCH	
Entrée: Healthy Choice Complete Meals Chicken Parmigiana	350
Side: Amy's Lentil Vegetable Soup (½ can)	160
Drink: Water	0
AFTERNOON SNACK	
Snack: Dole Fruit Crisps, Pineapple Mango (1 container)	150
Drink: Water	0
DINNER	
Vegetable: Dole Vegetable Medley (1 bag)	120
Entrée: Uncle Ben's Ready Whole Grain Medley Vegetable Harvest (1 package)	440
Side: Gorton's Grilled Garlic Butter Fish Fillet	100
Drink: Water	0
DESSERT	
Dessert: Skinny Cow Strawberry Shortcake Low Fat Ice Cream Sandwich	140
TOTAL	**2,030**

2,100-CALORIE MEAL PLAN	
	CALORIES
BREAKFAST	
Breakfast Entrée	300
Breakfast Side(s)	50
Drink	25
Total Breakfast calories	**375**
MORNING SNACK	
Morning Snack	150
Drink	25
Total Snack calories	**175**
LUNCH	
Fruit or Vegetable	50
Lunch Entrée	400
Lunch Side(s)	100
Drink	25
Total Lunch calories	**575**
AFTERNOON SNACK	
Total Snack calories	**150**
DINNER	
Fruit or Vegetable	100
Dinner Entrée	450
Dinner Side(s)	100
Drink	25
Total Dinner calories	**675**
DESSERT	
Total Dessert calories	**150**
TOTAL	**2,100**

SAMPLE 2,100-CALORIE MEAL PLAN	
	CALORIES
BREAKFAST	
Entrée: Nature's Path Organic Instant Hot Oatmeal Optimum Cinnamon Blueberry Flaxseed (2 packets)	300
Side: 8 large strawberries	46
Drink: Starbucks Tall Iced Coffee (sweetened)	60
MORNING SNACK	
Snack: Kashi TLC Chewy Granola Bar Peanut Peanut Butter	140
Drink: Water	0
LUNCH	
Entrée: Amy's Country Cheddar Bowl	430
Side: Campbell's Select Harvest Light Italian-Style Vegetable Microwave-able Bowl	100
Side: Mott's Plus Calcium Harvest Apple Sauce	50
Drink: Water	0
AFTERNOON SNACK	
Snack: Dole Fruit Crisps, Pineapple Mango (1 container)	150
Drink: Water	0
DINNER	
Vegetable: Green Giant Vegetable Medley (1 package)	120
Entrée: Burger King Tendergrill Chicken Sandwich on Ciabatta	470
Side: Campbell's Beefy Mushroom Condensed Soup (1 can)	125
Drink: Water	0
DESSERT	
Dessert: Keebler 100 Calorie Right Bites Mini Fudge Stripes	100
TOTAL	**2,091**

2,200-CALORIE MEAL PLAN

	CALORIES
BREAKFAST	
Breakfast Entrée	300
Breakfast Side(s)	100
Drink	25
Total Breakfast calories	**425**
MORNING SNACK	
Morning Snack	150
Drink	25
Total Snack calories	**175**
LUNCH	
Fruit or Vegetable	50
Lunch Entrée	400
Lunch Side(s)	100
Drink	25
Total Lunch calories	**575**
AFTERNOON SNACK	
Total Snack calories	**150**
DINNER	
Fruit or Vegetable	100
Dinner Entrée	450
Dinner Side(s)	150
Drink	25
Total Dinner calories	**725**
DESSERT	
Total Dessert calories	**150**
TOTAL	**2,200**

SAMPLE 2,200-CALORIE MEAL PLAN	CALORIES
BREAKFAST	
Entrée: Amy's Tofu Scramble	320
Side: Banana	105
Drink: Starbucks 16-Ounce Black Coffee	5
MORNING SNACK	
Snack: Amy's Cheese Pizza Toaster Pop	160
Drink: Water	0
LUNCH	
Fruit: 30 raspberries	30
Entrée: Lean Cuisine Casual Cuisine Deep Dish Three Meat Pizza	390
Side: Campbell's Healthy Request Chicken Noodle Condensed Soup (1 can)	175
Drink: Water	0
AFTERNOON SNACK	
Snack: Dole Fruit Crisps, Pineapple Mango (1 container)	150
Drink: Water	0
DINNER	
Entrée: Taco Bell ½ Pound Combo Burrito	460
Side: Taco Bell Mexican Rice	120
Vegetable: 1 medium tomato	22
Vegetable: 11 baby carrots	30
Vegetable: 1 large yellow pepper	50
Vegetable: Earthbound-Farms Organic Baby Romaine (1 package)	26
Side: Wishbone Salad Spritzers Balsamic Breeze Vinaigrette Dressing (10 sprays)	10
Drink: Water	0
DESSERT	
Dessert: Hershey's York Peppermint Pattie	140
	0
TOTAL	**2,193**

2,300-CALORIE MEAL PLAN

	CALORIES
BREAKFAST	
Breakfast Entrée	300
Breakfast Side(s)	100
Drink	25
Total Breakfast calories	**425**
MORNING SNACK	
Morning Snack	150
Drink	25
Total Snack calories	**175**
LUNCH	
Fruit or Vegetable	50
Lunch Entrée	400
Lunch Side(s)	150
Drink	25
Total Lunch calories	**625**
AFTERNOON SNACK	
Total Snack calories	**200**
DINNER	
Fruit or Vegetable	100
Dinner Entrée	450
Dinner Side(s)	150
Drink	25
Total Dinner calories	**725**
DESSERT	
Total Dessert calories	**150**
TOTAL	**2,300**

SAMPLE 2,300-CALORIE MEAL PLAN	CALORIES
BREAKFAST	
Entrée: McCann's Irish Oatmeal, Maple & Brown Sugar (2 packets)	320
Side: Banana	105
Drink: Starbucks Grande Black Coffee	5
MORNING SNACK	
Snack: Campbell's Creamy Chicken Soup at Hand	150
Drink: Water	0
LUNCH	
Entrée: Healthy Choice Fresh Mixers Sesame Teriyaki Chicken	380
Side: Organic Valley Provolone Cheese (1 slice)	70
Side: Amy's Light in Sodium Chunky Tomato Bisque Soup (½ can)	130
Drink: Water	0
AFTERNOON SNACK	
Snack: Yoplait Whips Strawberry Mist	140
Snack: Emerald 100 Calorie Packs Natural Walnuts and Almonds	100
Snack: 11 baby carrots	30
Drink: Water	0
DINNER	
Entrée: Bird's Eye Lightly Sauced Pasta Rigatoni & Vegetables with Tomato Parmesan Sauce	440
Vegetable: Ready Pac Spinach (1 bag)	40
Side: Dole Sugar Snap Peas (½ bag)	70
Side: Dr. Praeger's Sweet Potato Littles	60
Side: Gardenburger Portabella Veggie Burger	100
Drink: Water	0
DESSERT	
Dessert: Weight Watchers Turtle Sundae Ice Cream Cup	170
TOTAL	**2,310**

2,400-CALORIE MEAL PLAN	
	CALORIES
BREAKFAST	
Breakfast Entrée	350
Breakfast Side(s)	100
Drink	25
Total Breakfast calories	**475**
MORNING SNACK	
Morning Snack	200
Drink	25
Total Snack calories	**225**
LUNCH	
Fruit or Vegetable	50
Lunch Entrée	400
Lunch Side(s)	150
Drink	25
Total Lunch calories	**625**
AFTERNOON SNACK	
Total Snack calories	**200**
DINNER	
Fruit or Vegetable	100
Dinner Entrée	450
Dinner Side(s)	150
Drink	25
Total Dinner calories	**725**
DESSERT	
Total Dessert calories	**150**
TOTAL	**2,400**

SAMPLE 2,400-CALORIE MEAL PLAN	CALORIES
BREAKFAST	
Entrée: Starbucks Veggie, Egg and Monterey Jack Artisan Breakfast Sandwich	350
Side: Dole Peaches & Cream Parfait	120
Drink: Starbucks 16-Ounce Black Coffee	5
MORNING SNACK	
Snack: Campbell's Tomato Soup Microwaveable Bowl	200
Drink: Water	0
LUNCH	
Entrée: Annie Chun's Thai Peanut Noodle Express (1 container)	400
Side: Amy's Fat Free Chunky Vegetable Soup (½ can)	60
Side: Kraft Handi-Snacks Premium Breadsticks 'n Cheese Dip	110
Drink: Water	0
AFTERNOON SNACK	
Snack: Del Monte 100 Calorie Fruit Cocktail (1 can)	100
Snack: Emerald 100 Calorie Packs Natural Walnuts and Almonds	100
Drink: Water	0
DINNER	
Entrée: Olive Garden Seafood Brodetto	460
Side: Olive Garden Pasta e Fagioli Soup	130
Side: Olive Garden Breadstick (1)	150
Fruit: 1 cup blackberries	62
Drink: Water	0
DESSERT	
Dessert: Weight Watchers Ice Cream Candy Bar	150
TOTAL	**2,397**

2,500-CALORIE MEAL PLAN	
	CALORIES
BREAKFAST	
Breakfast Entrée	350
Breakfast Side(s)	100
Drink	25
Total Breakfast calories	475
MORNING SNACK	
Morning Snack	200
Drink	25
Total Snack calories	225
LUNCH	
Fruit or Vegetable	50
Lunch Entrée	400
Lunch Side(s)	150
Drink	25
Total Lunch calories	625
AFTERNOON SNACK	
Total Snack calories	250
DINNER	
Fruit or Vegetable	100
Dinner Entrée	500
Dinner Side(s)	150
Drink	25
Total Dinner calories	775
DESSERT	
Total Dessert calories	150
TOTAL	2,500

SAMPLE 2,500-CALORIE MEAL PLAN	CALORIES
BREAKFAST	
Entrée: Denny's 2 Scrambled Eggs & 4 Strips Bacon	380
Side: Del Monte 100 Calorie Pear Halves (1 can)	100
Drink: Black coffee (12 ounces)	5
MORNING SNACK	
Snack: Healthy Choice Microwaveable Bowls Cheese Tortellini	180
Fruit: Kiwi	52
Drink: Water	0
LUNCH	
Fruit: 8 large strawberries	46
Entrée: Chef Boyardee Mini Ravioli Microwaveable Big Size Bowl	384
Side: Hormel Hard Salami (6 slices)	110
Drink: Water	0
AFTERNOON SNACK	
Snack: Lean Cuisine Cafe Cuisine Fiesta Grilled Chicken	260
Fruit: 4 5-inch celery stalks	12
Drink: Water	0
DINNER	
Vegetable: Birds Eye Steamfresh Premium Selects Broccoli Florets (1 bag)	120
Entrée: Amy's Cheese Enchilada	480
Side: Perdue Buffalo Style Chicken Strips (3 strips)	210
Drink: Water	0
DESSERT	
Dessert: Skinny Cow Chocolate Peanut Butter Low Fat Ice Cream Sandwich	150
TOTAL	**2,489**

BUILD-A-MEAL

Build-a-Meal Foods

DIET DETECTIVE'S WHAT YOU NEED TO KNOW

REMEMBER TO EAT YOUR FRUITS AND VEGETABLES

Want to stay full longer? Enjoy a fruit or vegetable for your [SIDE OR SNACK, DEPENDING ON WHICH LIST] instead. In addition to all the nutrients and health-promoting compounds in fruits and vegetables, they also contain fiber, which helps fill you up so you eat less—and lose weight. See pages 167 and 170 for fruit and vegetable options.

Look for these symbols if you're interested in the following food choices:

Low Carb =

Sodium Controlled =

Vegetarian =

DIET DETECTIVE'S WHAT YOU NEED TO KNOW

CALORIE RANGES

While the following lists are separated into calorie categories, they are actually calorie ranges. So, for example, the 250-calorie vegetables may actually have between 250 and 299 calories.

Build-a-Meal
250-Calorie Breakfast Entrées

Low Carb= 🍞 **Sodium Controlled=** 🧂 **Vegetarian=** 🌿

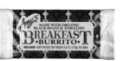

AMY'S
Breakfast Burrito
1 burrito
270 Calories
🌿

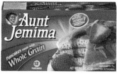

AUNT JEMIMA
Pancakes Made with
Whole Grain
3 pancakes
240 Calories
🧂 🌿

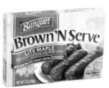

BANQUET
Brown 'N Serve Lite
Maple Sausage Links
6 links
240 Calories
🍞

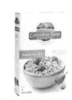

CASCADIAN FARM
Honey Nut O's with Skim
Milk
⅔ cup + ½ cup
253 Calories
🧂 🌿

CLIF
Black Cherry Almond
1 bar
240 Calories
🧂 🌿

CLIF
Chocolate Chip
1 bar
240 Calories
🧂 🌿

GENERAL MILLS
Cocoa Puffs (mini box
from variety pack)
2 mini boxes
260 Calories
🧂 🌿

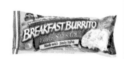

JOSÉ OLÉ
Breakfast Burrito, Egg &
Sausage
1 burrito
270 Calories

KASHI
GoLean Crunch! Cereal
Honey Almond Flax with
Skim Milk
1 cup + ½ cup
243 Calories
🧂 🌿

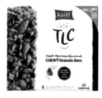

KASHI
TLC Chewy Granola Bars,
Dark Mocha Almond
2 bars
260 Calories
🧂 🌿

KASHI
TLC Fruit & Grain Bars,
Cranberry Walnut
2 bars
240 Calories
🧂 🌿

KELLOGG'S
Mini Wheats Cereal
in a Cup
1 container
240 Calories
🧂 🌿

Build-a-Meal
250-Calorie Breakfast Entrées

Low Carb=   Sodium Controlled=   Vegetarian=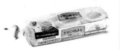

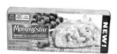

MORNINGSTAR FARMS
Bacon Egg & Cheese
Biscuits
1 biscuit
270 Calories

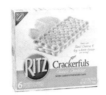

NABISCO
Ritz Crackerfuls, Classic
Cheddar
2 packages
260 Calories

NATURE'S PATH
Organic Toaster Pastries,
Blueberry
1 pastry
240 Calories

NATURE'S PATH
EnviroKidz Organic Crispy
Rice Cereal Bars, Peanut
Choco Drizzle
2 bars
240 Calories

PLANTERS
Nut-rition Heart Healthy
Mix Bags
1 bag
250 Calories

POST
Grape-Nuts Cereal
with Skim Milk
½ cup + ½ cup
240 Calories

POST
Shredded Wheat Wheat
'N Bran with Skim Milk
1¼ cup + ½ cup
240 Calories

THOMAS'
100% Whole Wheat
Hearty Muffins
2 muffins
240 Calories

THOMAS'
Mini Bagels, Blueberry
2 mini bagels
249 Calories

THOMAS'
Blueberry Bagels
1 bagel
270 Calories

Build-a-Meal
300-Calorie Breakfast Entrées

Low Carb= **Sodium Controlled=** 🧂 **Vegetarian=** 🥕

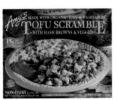

AMY'S
Tofu Scramble
1 container
320 Calories

BARBARA'S
Puffins Peanut Butter
Cereal with Skim Milk
1½ cup + 1 cup
306 Calories

BEAR NAKED
Fruit and Nut Granola
2-ounce bag
280 Calories

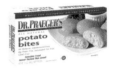

DR. PRAEGER'S
Potato Bites
6 pieces
330 Calories

GENERAL MILLS
Golden Grahams (mini
box from variety pack)
2 mini boxes
280 Calories

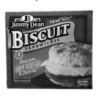

JIMMY DEAN
Biscuit Sandwiches,
Bacon Egg & Cheese
1 sandwich
320 Calories

KASHI
GoLean Crunch! Cereal
with Skim Milk
1 cup + 1 cup
280 Calories

KASHI
TLC Chewy Granola Bars,
Honey Almond Flax
2 bars
280 Calories

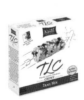

KASHI
TLC Chewy Granola Bars,
Trail Mix
2 bars
280 Calories

KASHI
GoLean Hearty All Natural
Instant Hot Cereal with
Clusters, Honey & Cin-
namon
2 packets
300 Calories

KASHI
Heart to Heart Instant
Oatmeal, Golden Brown
Maple
2 packets
320 Calories

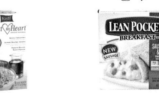

LEAN POCKETS
Breakfast Sausage Egg &
Cheese
1 piece
280 Calories

Build-a-Meal
300-Calorie Breakfast Entrées

Low Carb=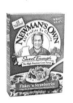 Sodium Controlled= Vegetarian=

LEAN POCKETS
Breakfast Applewood
Bacon Egg & Cheese
1 piece
290 Calories
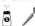

MCCANN'S
Irish Oatmeal, Maple &
Brown Sugar
2 packets
320 Calories

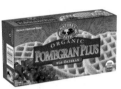

NATURE'S PATH
Organic Pomegran Plus
with Oatbran Waffles
4 waffles
320 Calories

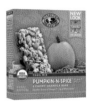

NATURE'S PATH
Organic Chewy Granola
Bars, Pumpkin-N-Spice
2 bars
280 Calories

NATURE'S PATH
Organic Instant Hot Oat-
meal Optimum Cinnamon
Blueberry Flaxseed
2 packets
300 Calories

NEWMAN'S OWN
Flakes 'n Strawberries
with Skim Milk
1½ cup + 1 cup
300 Calories

POST
Banana Nut Crunch with
Skim Milk
1 cup + ½ cup
280 Calories

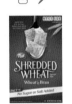

POST
Wheat 'n Bran Shredded
Wheat with Skim Milk
1¼ cups + 1 cup
280 Calories

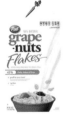

POST
Grape-Nuts Flakes with
Skim Milk
1½ cup + 1 cup
300 Calories

POST
Honey Bunches of Oats
with Skim Milk
1½ cups + 1 cup
320 Calories

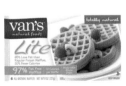

VAN'S
Lite Waffles
4 waffles
280 Calories

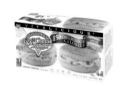

VITALICIOUS
Egg 'n Cheese with
Veggies VitaSandwich
2 sandwiches
300 Calories

Build-a-Meal
350-Calorie Breakfast Entrées

Low Carb= **Sodium Controlled=** **Vegetarian=**

EMERALD
Breakfast on the Go,
Berry Nut Blend
2 pouches
360 Calories

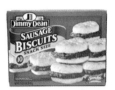

JIMMY DEAN
Sausage Biscuit
Snack Size
1 sandwich
360 Calories

KASHI
GoLean Cereal
with Skim Milk
2 cups + 1 cup
366 Calories

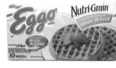

KELLOGG'S
Eggo Nutri-Grain Whole
Wheat Waffles
4 waffles
340 Calories

LUNA
Protein Cookie Dough
2 bars
360 Calories

NATURE'S PATH
Organic Instant Hot
Oatmeal, Multigrain
Raisin Spice
2 packets
360 Calories

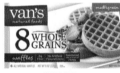

VAN'S
Multigrain Waffles
4 waffles
360 Calories

Build-a-Meal
400-Calorie Breakfast Entrées

Low Carb= 🍞 **Sodium Controlled=** 🧂 **Vegetarian=** 🍴

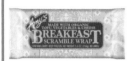
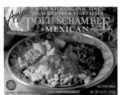

AMY'S
Breakfast Scramble Wrap
1 wrap
380 Calories

AMY'S
Mexican Tofu Scramble
1 container
400 Calories
🍴

DEL MONTE
SunFresh Citrus Salad
1 jar
400 Calories
🧂 🍴

EMERALD
Breakfast on the Go
S'mores
2 pouches
400 Calories
🧂 🍴

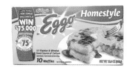

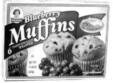

KASHI
GoLean Crisp! Cereal
Toasted Berry Crumble
with Skim Milk
1½ cups + 1 cup
390 Calories

🧂 🍴

KELLOGG'S
Eggo Homestyle Waffles
4 waffles
380 Calories
🍴

KELLOGG'S
Pop-Tarts, Strawberry
2 pastries
400 Calories
🍴

LITTLE DEBBIE
Blueberry Muffins
2 muffins
380 Calories
🧂 🍴

NATURE'S PATH
Organic Instant Hot
Oatmeal, Original
2 packets
380 Calories

🧂 🍴

NATURE'S PATH
Organic Instant Hot
Oatmeal, Apple Cinnamon
2 packets
380 Calories
🧂 🍴

NATURE'S PATH
Organic Frosted Toaster
Pastries, Blueberry
2 pastries
400 Calories

🧂 🍴

NATURE'S PATH
Organic Instant Hot
Oatmeal, Maple Nut
2 packets
410 Calories

🧂 🍴

Build-a-Meal
400-Calorie Breakfast Entrées

Low Carb= **Sodium Controlled=** **Vegetarian=**

NATURE'S PATH
Organic Instant Hot Oat-
meal Flax Plus
2 packets
420 Calories

NATURE'S PATH
Frosted Raspberry
Toaster Pastries
2 pastries
420 Calories

POST
Shredded Wheat with
Skim Milk
2 cups + 1 cup
420 Calories

SMART ONES
Morning Express
Canadian Style Bacon
English Muffin Sandwich
2 sandwiches
420 Calories

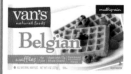

VAN'S
Multigrain Belgian Waffles
4 waffles
380 Calories

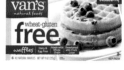

VAN'S
Blueberry Wheat & Gluten
Free Waffles
4 waffles
420 Calories

Build-a-Meal 50-Calorie Breakfast Sides and Morning Snacks

Low Carb= 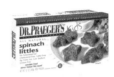 **Sodium Controlled=** **Vegetarian=**

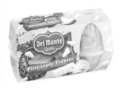

DEL MONTE
Pineapple Tidbits
1 container
70 Calories

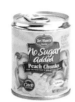

DEL MONTE
No Sugar Added Peach
Chunks
1 8.14-ounce can
60 Calories

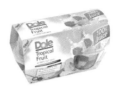

DOLE
Tropical Fruit
1 container
60 Calories

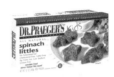

DR. PRAEGER'S
Spinach Littles
2 pieces
45 Calories

EARTH'S BEST
Organic Yogurt Rice Crisp
Bars, Vanilla
1 bar
70 Calories

EARTH'S BEST
Sunny Days Snack Bars,
Apple
1 bar
70 Calories

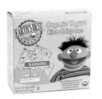

EARTH'S BEST
Organic Yogurt Rice Crisp
Bars, Banana
1 bar
70 Calories

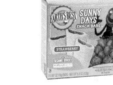

EARTH'S BEST
Sunny Days Snack Bars,
Strawberry
1 bar
70 Calories

THE LAUGHING COW
Light Mozzarella, Sun-
Dried Tomato & Basil
1 wedge
35 Calories

MOTT'S
Healthy Harvest No Sugar
Added Granny Smith
Apple Sauce
1 4-ounce container
50 Calories

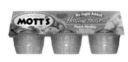

MOTT'S
Healthy Harvest No Sugar
Added Peach Medley
Apple Sauce
1 4-ounce container
50 Calories

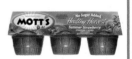

MOTT'S
Healthy Harvest No Sugar
Added Summer Straw-
berry Apple Sauce
1 4-ounce container
50 Calories

Build-a-Meal 50-Calorie
Breakfast Sides and Morning Snacks

Low Carb= Sodium Controlled= Vegetarian=

MOTT'S
No Sugar Added Natural
Apple Sauce
1 4-ounce container
50 Calories

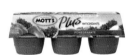

MOTT'S
Plus Antioxidants Pome-
granate Apple Sauce
1 4-ounce container
50 Calories

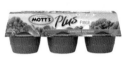

MOTT'S
Plus Fiber No Sugar
Added Cranberry Rasp-
berry Apple Sauce
1 4-ounce container
50 Calories

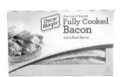

OSCAR MAYER
Fully Cooked Bacon
4 slices
70 Calories

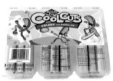

READY PAC
Celery with Ranch Dip
Snack Pac
1 package
60 Calories

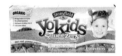

STONYFIELD
YoKids Squeezers,
Strawberry
1 tube
50 Calories

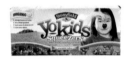

STONYFIELD
YoKids Squeezers,
Cherry & Berry
1 tube
60 Calories

**STRETCH ISLAND
FRUIT CO.**
All-Natural Fruit Strip,
Mango Sunrise
1 strip
45 Calories

SUNSWEET
60 Calorie Packs Prunes
1 pouch
60 Calories

SUNSWEET
70 Calorie Packs Dried
Apricots
1 pouch
70 Calories

YOPLAIT
Simply Go-Gurt,
Strawberry
1 tube
70 Calories

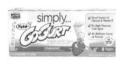

ALL-AMERICAN DIET

Build-a-Meal 100-Calorie Breakfast Sides and Morning Snacks

Low Carb= Sodium Controlled= Vegetarian=

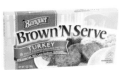

BANQUET
Brown 'N Serve Turkey
Sausage Patties
2 patties
100 Calories

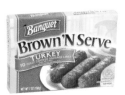

BANQUET
Brown 'N Serve Turkey
Sausage Links
3 links
110 Calories

BLUE DIAMOND
100 Calorie Packs Whole
Almonds Natural
1 bag
100 Calories

BREAKSTONE'S
4% Milkfat Cottage
Cheese Snack Size
1 4-ounce container
110 Calories

BREAKSTONE'S
Cottage Doubles,
Pineapple
1 container
130 Calories

BREAKSTONE'S
Cottage Doubles,
Strawberry
1 container
130 Calories

CAMPBELL'S
Chicken with Mini
Noodles Soup at Hand
1 container
80 Calories

CASCADIAN FARM
Dark Chocolate Almond
Granola Bars
1 bar
130 Calories

CHOBANI
Nonfat Greek Yogurt,
Vanilla
1 container
120 Calories

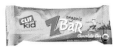

CLIF KID
ZBar, Chocolate Chip
1 bar
130 Calories

DANNON
Light & Fit Lemon Chiffon
1 container
80 Calories

DANNON
Light & Fit Cherry Vanilla
1 container
80 Calories

Build-a-Meal 100-Calorie Breakfast Sides and Morning Snacks

Low Carb= **Sodium Controlled=** 🧂 **Vegetarian=** 🌿

DEL MONTE
100 Calorie Pear Halves
1 can
100 Calories

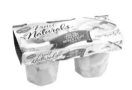

DEL MONTE
Fruit Naturals Cherry Mixed Fruit
1 8-ounce cup
120 Calories

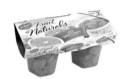

DEL MONTE
Fruit Naturals Red Grape-fruit
1 8-ounce cup
120 Calories

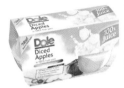

DOLE
Diced Apples
1 container
80 Calories

DOLE
Real Fruit Bites with Yogurt and Whole Grain Oats Mango Chunks
1 pouch
80 Calories

DOLE
Real Fruit Bites with Yogurt and Whole Grain Oats Pineapple Chunks
1 pouch
80 Calories

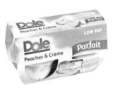

DOLE
Peaches & Cream Parfait
1 container
120 Calories

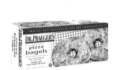

DR. PRAEGER'S
Pizza Bagels
1 piece
110 Calories

EARTH'S BEST
Organic Letter of the Day Cookies, Very Vanilla
1 pouch
100 Calories

EMERALD
100 Calorie Packs Cocoa Roast Almonds
1 pouch
100 Calories

EMERALD
100 Calorie Packs Cinnamon Roast Almonds
1 pouch
100 Calories

ENTENMANN'S
100 Calorie Blueberry Muffins
1 muffin
100 Calories

ALL-AMERICAN DIET

74

Build-a-Meal 100-Calorie
Breakfast Sides and Morning Snacks

Low Carb= Sodium Controlled= Vegetarian=

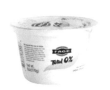

FAGE
Total 0% Nonfat Greek
Yogurt
1 container
90 Calories

GENERAL MILLS
Cheerios
1 mini box
100 Calories

GENERAL MILLS
Honey Nut Cheerios
1 mini box
120 Calories

GENERAL MILLS
Frosted Cheerios
1 mini box
120 Calories

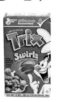

GENERAL MILLS
Trix
1 mini box
120 Calories

GENERAL MILLS
Lucky Charms
1 mini box
130 Calories

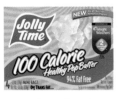

JOLLY TIME
100 Calorie Healthy Pop
Butter
1 bag
90 Calories

KASHI
TLC Soft-Baked Cereal
Bars, Baked Apple Spice
1 bar
110 Calories

KASHI
TLC Soft-Baked Cereal
Bars, Ripe Strawberry
1 bar
110 Calories

KASHI
TLC Soft-Baked Cereal
Bars, Blackberry Graham
1 bar
110 Calories

KASHI
TLC Chewy Granola Bars,
Cherry Dark Chocolate
1 bar
120 Calories

KASHI
TLC Fruit & Grain Bars,
Dark Chocolate Coconut
1 bar
120 Calories

75

BREAKFAST SIDES AND MORNING SNACKS

Build-a-Meal 100-Calorie
Breakfast Sides and Morning Snacks

Low Carb= 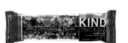 **Sodium Controlled=** **Vegetarian=**

KIND
Fruit & Nut Bars, Apple
Cinnamon & Pecan
1 bar
90 Calories

MCCANN'S
Irish Oatmeal, Regular
1 packet
100 Calories

NATURE'S PATH
EnviroKidz Organic
Crispy Rice Cereal Bars,
Chocolate
1 bar
110 Calories

NATURE'S PATH
EnviroKidz Organic Crispy
Rice Cereal Bars,
Peanut Butter
1 bar
110 Calories

NATURE'S PATH
EnviroKidz Organic Crispy
Rice Cereal Bars,
Berry Blast
1 bar
110 Calories

NATURE'S PATH
EnviroKidz Organic Crispy
Rice Cereal Bars,
Fruity Burst
1 bar
110 Calories

OCEAN SPRAY
100 Calorie Packs
Craisins
1 pouch
100 Calories

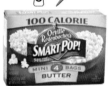

**ORVILLE
REDENBACHER'S**
Smart Pop Butter
Mini Bags
1 mini bag
110 Calories

PAPETTI FOODS
Quick Whites 100%
Liquid Egg Whites
1 cup
120 Calories

PEPPERIDGE FARM
100 Calorie Pouches
Goldfish, Pretzel
1 pouch
100 Calories

PIRATE'S BOOTY
Barbeque Rice and Corn
Puffs
1-ounce bag
130 Calories

PRINGLES
Baked Wheat Stix, Honey
Butter
1 package
90 Calories

Build-a-Meal 100-Calorie
Breakfast Sides and Morning Snacks

Low Carb= **Sodium Controlled=** **Vegetarian=**

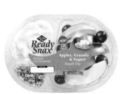

READY PAC
Ready Snax Apples,
Granola & Yogurt Snack
Pac
1 package
100 Calories

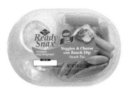

READY PAC
Ready Snax Veggies &
Cheese with Ranch Dip
Snack Pac
1 package
130 Calories

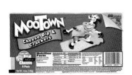

SARGENTO
MooTown Cheese Dip &
Crackers
1 package
100 Calories

SNACK PACK
Juicy Gels, Strawberry
1 cup
100 Calories

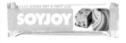

SOYJOY
Baked Whole Soy & Fruit
Bar, Banana
1 bar
130 Calories

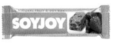

SOYJOY
All Natural Fruit & Soy Bar,
Strawberry
1 bar
130 Calories

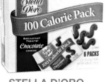

STELLA D'ORO
Breakfast Treats
Chocolate Cookies
1 pouch
100 Calories

STONYFIELD
0% Fat Plain Smooth and
Creamy
1 container
80 Calories

STONYFIELD
Low Fat Plain Smooth
and Creamy
1 container
90 Calories

STONYFIELD
YoBaby Whole Milk,
Blueberry
1 container
100 Calories

STONYFIELD
YoBaby Whole Milk,
Banana
1 container
100 Calories

STONYFIELD
Oikos Greek Yogurt,
Blueberry
1 container
120 Calories

Build-a-Meal 100-Calorie Breakfast Sides and Morning Snacks

Low Carb= **Sodium Controlled=** **Vegetarian=**

STONYFIELD
Low Fat Cherry Vanilla
Smooth and Creamy
1 container
130 Calories

**STRETCH ISLAND
FRUIT CO.**
Fruitabü Smooshed Apple
1 roll
80 Calories

**STRETCH ISLAND
FRUIT CO.**
All-Natural Fruit Strip,
Harvest Grape
1 strip
90 Calories

SUN-MAID
Raisins
1 1.5-ounce box
90 Calories

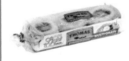

THOMAS'
Light Multi-Grain
Hearty Muffins
1 muffin
100 Calories

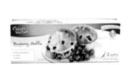

THOMAS'
Bagel Thins, Everything
1 thin
110 Calories

VITALICIOUS
Sugar Free Banana
Nut VitaTops
1 muffin
90 Calories

WEIGHT WATCHERS
Vanilla Nonfat Yogurt
1 container
100 Calories

WEIGHT WATCHERS
Apple Pie a la Mode
Nonfat Yogurt
1 container
100 Calories

WEIGHT WATCHERS
Blueberry Muffins
1 muffin
100 Calories

YOPLAIT
Low Fat Thick & Creamy
Strawberry
1 container
100 Calories

YOPLAIT
Light Very Vanilla
1 container
110 Calories

Build-a-Meal 150-Calorie Breakfast Sides and Morning Snacks

Low Carb= 🍞 **Sodium Controlled=** 🧂 **Vegetarian=** 🌿

AMY'S
Summer Corn and Vegetable Soup
½ can
150 Calories
🌿

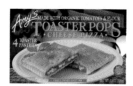

AMY'S
Cheese Pizza Toaster Pops
1 piece
160 Calories
🧂 🌿

AMY'S
Hot Cereal Cream of Rice Bowl
1 bowl
170 Calories
🧂 🌿

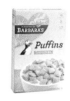

BARBARA'S
Puffins Original Cereal with Skim Milk
¾ cup + ½ cup
133 Calories
🧂 🌿

CAMPBELL'S
Chicken Noodle Microwaveable Bowl
1 bowl
140 Calories

CAMPBELL'S
Creamy Chicken Soup at Hand
1 container
150 Calories

CAMPBELL'S
Chicken Noodle Condensed Soup
1 can
150 Calories

CAMPBELL'S
New England Clam Chowder Soup at Hand
1 container
150 Calories
🍞

CAMPBELL'S
Healthy Kids Chicken & Stars Condensed Soup
1 can
161 Calories

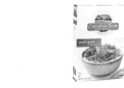

CASCADIAN FARM
Multi Grain with Skim Milk
¾ cup + ½ cup
153 Calories
🧂 🌿

CASCADIAN FARM
Sweet and Salty Peanut Pretzel Chewy Granola Bars
1 bar
160 Calories
🧂 🌿

CHOBANI
Nonfat Greek Yogurt, Raspberry
1 container
140 Calories
🧂 🌿

Build-a-Meal 150-Calorie Breakfast Sides and Morning Snacks

Low Carb= **Sodium Controlled=**  **Vegetarian=**

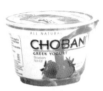

CHOBANI
Nonfat Greek Yogurt,
Strawberry
1 container
140 Calories

CHOBANI
Lowfat Greek Yogurt,
Pineapple
1 container
160 Calories

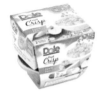

DOLE
Fruit Crisps, Apple Pear
1 container
150 Calories

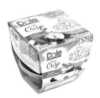

DOLE
Fruit Crisps, Apple
Cinnamon
1 container
160 Calories

EARTH'S BEST
Yummy Tummy Oatmeal
Maple & Brown Sugar
1 packet
160 Calories

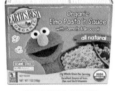

EARTH'S BEST
Organic Elmo
Pasta 'n Sauce
1 meal
160 Calories

GENERAL MILLS
Cinnamon Toast Crunch
(mini box from
variety pack)
1 mini box
170 Calories

KASHI
GoLean Creamy All
Natural Instant Hot
Cereal, Truly Vanilla
1 packet
150 Calories

KASHI
TLC Chewy Granola Bars,
Peanut Peanut Butter
1 bar
140 Calories

KASHI
7-Grain Waffles
2 waffles
150 Calories

KASHI
GoLean Crunchy Protein
& Fiber Bar, Chocolate
Caramel
1 bar
150 Calories

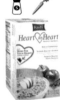

KASHI
Heart to Heart Instant
Oatmeal, Apple Cinnamon
1 packet
160 Calories

ALL-AMERICAN DIET

Build-a-Meal 150-Calorie
Breakfast Sides and Morning Snacks

Low Carb= **Sodium Controlled=** **Vegetarian=**

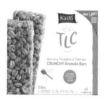

KASHI
TLC Crunchy Granola
Bars, Honey Toasted
7 Grain
2 bars
170 Calories
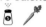

KELLOGG'S
Special K Original cereal
in a Cup
1 container
140 Calories

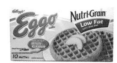

KELLOGG'S
Eggo Nutri-Grain Low
Fat Waffles
2 waffles
140 Calories

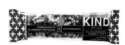

KIND
Plus Bars, Pomegranate
Blueberry Pistachio +
Antioxidants
1 bar
170 Calories

LENDER'S BAGELS
Plain Original Freezer
Bagels
1 bagel
140 Calories

RITZ
Crackerfuls, Four Cheese
1 package
130 Calories

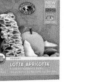

NATURE'S PATH
Organic Chewy Granola
Bars, Lotta' Apricotta
1 bar
140 Calories

NATURE'S PATH
Organic Chewy Granola
Bars, Sunny Hemp
1 bar
140 Calories

NATURE'S PATH
Organic Instant Hot Oat-
meal Optimum, Cranberry
Ginger
1 packet
150 Calories

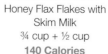

NEWMAN'S OWN
Honey Flax Flakes with
Skim Milk
¾ cup + ½ cup
140 Calories

PLANTERS
Nut-rition Heart Healthy
Bars
1 bar
160 Calories

POST
Shredded Wheat
2 biscuits
160 Calories

81

Build-a-Meal 150-Calorie
Breakfast Sides and Morning Snacks

Low Carb= **Sodium Controlled=** **Vegetarian=**

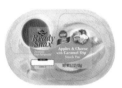

READY PAC
Ready Snax Apples &
Cheese with Caramel Dip
Snack Pac
1 package
140 Calories

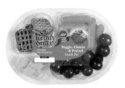

READY PAC
Ready Snax Veggie,
Cheese & Pretzel Snack
Pac
1 package
150 Calories

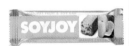

SOYJOY
All Natural Fruit & Soy Bar,
Apple Walnut
1 bar
140 Calories

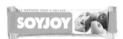

SOYJOY
All Natural Fruit & Soy Bar,
Mango Coconut
1 bar
140 Calories

STONYFIELD
Super Smoothie,
Strawberry
1 6-ounce bottle
140 Calories

VAN'S
Chocolate Chip Mini
Waffles
8 mini waffles
150 Calories

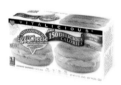

VITALICIOUS
Egg 'n Cheese
VitaSandwiches
1 sandwich
150 Calories

WEIGHT WATCHERS
Original Plain Bagels
1 bagel
150 Calories

YOPLAIT
Original Strawberry
Banana
1 container
170 Calories

YOPLAIT
Original French Vanilla
1 container
170 Calories

Build-a-Meal 200-Calorie
Breakfast Sides and Morning Snacks

Low Carb=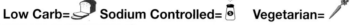 Sodium Controlled= Vegetarian=

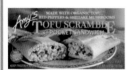

AMY'S
Tofu Scramble in a Pocket
Sandwich
1 sandwich
180 Calories

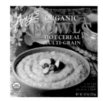

AMY'S
Hot Cereal Multi Grain
Bowl
1 bowl
190 Calories

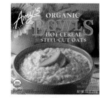

AMY'S
Hot Cereal Steel-Cut Oats
Bowl
1 bowl
220 Calories

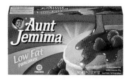

AUNT JEMIMA
Low Fat Pancakes
3 pancakes
200 Calories

CAMPBELL'S
98% Fat Free Broccoli
Cheese Condensed Soup
1 can
175 Calories

CAMPBELL'S
Cream of Mushroom with
Roasted Garlic
Condensed Soup
1 can
175 Calories

CAMPBELL'S
Light Chicken Gumbo
Condensed Soup
1 can
175 Calories

CAMPBELL'S
Chicken Vegetable
Condensed Soup
1 can
200 Calories

CAMPBELL'S
Healthy Request Select
Harvest Italian-Style
Wedding Soup
1 can
200 Calories

CAMPBELL'S
Tomato Soup
Microwaveable Bowl
1 bowl
200 Calories

CAMPBELL'S
Select Harvest Chicken
with Egg Noodles
Microwaveable Bowl
1 bowl
220 Calories

CAMPBELL'S
Healthy Request Chicken
Noodle Chunky Soup
1 can
220 Calories

BREAKFAST SIDES AND MORNING SNACKS

Build-a-Meal 200-Calorie Breakfast Sides and Morning Snacks

Low Carb= **Sodium Controlled=** **Vegetarian=**

CAMPBELL'S
Beef with Vegetables &
Barley Condensed Soup
1 can
225 Calories

CAMPBELL'S
Minestrone Condensed
Soup
1 can
225 Calories

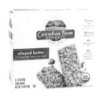

CASCADIAN FARM
Almond Butter Crunchy
Granola Bars
2 bars
180 Calories

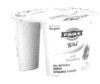

FAGE
Total with Strawberry
Greek Yogurt
1 container
210 Calories

FRESH EXPRESS
Waldorf Chicken Gourmet
Café Salad
1 container
180 Calories

GENERAL MILLS
Cheerios Cereal in a Cup
1 container
200 Calories

HEALTHY CHOICE
Microwaveable Bowls
Cheese Tortellini
1 bowl
180 Calories

JIMMY DEAN
D-Lights Canadian Bacon
Honey Wheat Muffin
1 sandwich
230 Calories

JIMMY DEAN
D-Lights Turkey Bacon
Bowl
1 bowl
230 Calories

JIMMY DEAN
D-Lights Turkey Sausage
Bowl
1 bowl
230 Calories

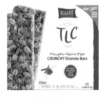

KASHI
TLC Crunchy Granola
Bars, Pumpkin Spice Flax
2 bars
180 Calories

KASHI
7 Whole Grain Puffs Cereal with Skim Milk
2 cups + 1 cup
220 Calories

ALL-AMERICAN DIET

Build-a-Meal 200-Calorie
Breakfast Sides and Morning Snacks

Low Carb=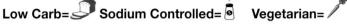 Sodium Controlled= Vegetarian=

KASHI
Go Lean Crisp! Toasted
Berry Crumble
with Skim Milk
1 cup + ½ cup
223 Calories

KELLOGG'S
Frosted Flakes Cereal
in a Cup
1 container
220 Calories

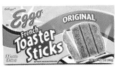

KELLOGG'S
Eggo French Toaster
Sticks
2 pieces
220 Calories

KELLOGG'S
Smart Start Original
Antioxidants Strong Heart
Cereal with Skim Milk
1 cup + ½ cup
230 Calories

KIND
Fruit & Nut Bars, Peanut
Butter & Strawberry
1 bar
190 Calories

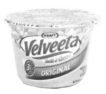

KRAFT
Velveeta Shells & Cheese
Original Cup
1 container
220 Calories

LEAN CUISINE
Spa Cuisine Szechuan-
Style Stir Fry with Shrimp
1 meal
210 Calories

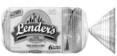

LENDER'S BAGELS
100% Whole Wheat Origi-
nal Freezer Bagels
1 bagel
180 Calories

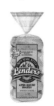

LENDER'S BAGELS
Cinnamon Raisin Swirl
Bagel Shop Bagels
1 bagel
180 Calories

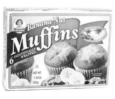

LENDER'S BAGELS
100% Whole Wheat New
York Style Bagels
1 bagel
210 Calories

LITTLE DEBBIE
Banana Nut Muffins
1 muffin
210 Calories

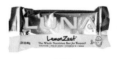

LUNA
Lemon Zest
1 bar
180 Calories

BREAKFAST SIDES AND MORNING SNACKS

Build-a-Meal 200-Calorie Breakfast Sides and Morning Snacks

Low Carb= **Sodium Controlled=** **Vegetarian=**

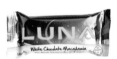

LUNA
White Chocolate Macadamia
1 bar
190 Calories

NATURE'S PATH
Organic Frosted Toaster Pastries, Apple Cinnamon
1 pastry
210 Calories

NATURE'S PATH
Organic Frosted Toaster Pastries, Brown Sugar Maple Cinnamon
1 pastry
210 Calories

NATURE'S PATH
Organic Frosted Toaster Pastries, Cherry Pomegran
1 pastry
210 Calories

NATURE'S PATH
Organic Frosted Toaster Pastries, Chocolate
1 pastry
210 Calories

POST
Shredded Wheat Honey Nut with Skim Milk
1 cup + ½ cup
220 Calories

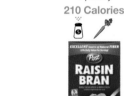

POST
Raisin Bran with Skim Milk
1 cup + ½ cup
230 Calories

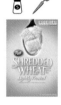

POST
Shredded Wheat Lightly Frosted with Skim Milk
1 cup + ½ cup
240 Calories

QUAKER
Express Oatmeal Cup, Baked Apple
1 container
200 Calories

QUAKER
Express Oatmeal Cup, Golden Brown Sugar
1 container
200 Calories

QUAKER
Express Oatmeal Cup, Cinnamon Roll
1 container
200 Calories

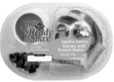

READY PAC
Apples, Celery, Raisins with Peanut Butter Snack Pac
1 package
210 Calories

Build-a-Meal 200-Calorie
Breakfast Sides and Morning Snacks

Low Carb= **Sodium Controlled=**  **Vegetarian=**

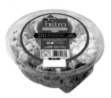

READY PAC
Chicken Cranberry Walnut
Bistro Salad
1 package
210 Calories

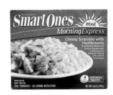

SMART ONES
Morning Express Cheesy
Scramble with Hash-
browns
1 meal
210 Calories

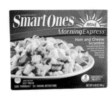

SMART ONES
Morning Express Ham &
Cheese Scramble
1 meal
220 Calories

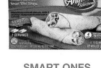

SMART ONES
Chicken Ranchero Smart
Mini Wraps
2 wraps
220 Calories

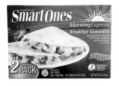

SMART ONES
Morning Express Break-
fast Quesadilla
1 piece
230 Calories

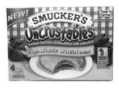

SMUCKER'S
Uncrustables Peanut But-
ter and Strawberry Jam
on Whole Wheat Bread
1 sandwich
210 Calories

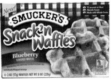

SMUCKER'S
Snack'n Waffles,
Blueberry
1 waffle
220 Calories

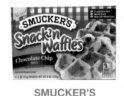

SMUCKER'S
Snack'n Waffles,
Chocolate Chip
1 waffle
220 Calories

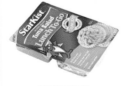

STARKIST
Tuna Salad Lunch To-Go
Chunk Light
1 kit
210 Calories

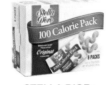

STELLA D'ORo
Breakfast Treats Original
Cookies
2 pouches
200 Calories

STONYFIELD
0% Fat Chocolate
Underground
1 container
180 Calories

STONYFIELD
Super Smoothie,
Raspberry
1 10-ounce bottle
230 Calories

Build-a-Meal 200-Calorie Breakfast Sides and Morning Snacks

Low Carb= **Sodium Controlled=** **Vegetarian=**

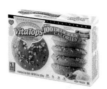

STONYFIELD
Super Smoothie, Peach
1 10-ounce bottle
230 Calories

VITALICIOUS
Banana Nut VitaTops
2 muffins
200 Calories

VITALICIOUS
Deep & Velvety Chocolate
VitaBrownie
2 muffins
200 Calories

YOPLAIT
Thick & Creamy Vanilla
1 container
180 Calories

Build-a-Meal
300-Calorie Lunch Entrées

Low Carb= 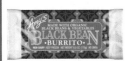 **Sodium Controlled=** **Vegetarian=**

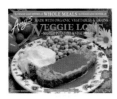

AMY'S
Black Bean Vegetable
Burrito
1 burrito
280 Calories

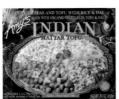

AMY'S
Indian Mattar Tofu
1 meal
280 Calories

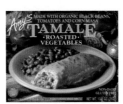

AMY'S
Roasted Vegetables
Tamale
1 meal
280 Calories

AMY'S
Spicy Chili
½ can
280 Calories

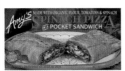

AMY'S
Spinach Pizza in a Pocket
Sandwich
1 sandwich
280 Calories

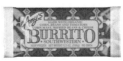

AMY'S
Southwestern Burrito
1 burrito
290 CALORIES

AMY'S
Brown Rice with
Black-Eyed Peas
and Veggies Bowl
1 bowl
290 Calories

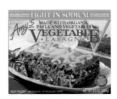

AMY'S
Light in Sodium Vegetable
Lasagna
1 container
290 Calories

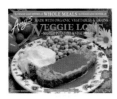

AMY'S
Whole Meals Veggie Loaf
1 meal
290 Calories

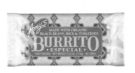

AMY'S
Burrito Especial
1 burrito
300 Calories

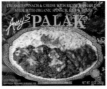

AMY'S
Indian Palak Paneer
1 container
300 Calories

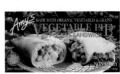

AMY'S
Vegetable Pie in a Pocket
Sandwich
1 sandwich
300 Calories

Build-a-Meal
300-Calorie Lunch Entrées

Low Carb= 🍞 Sodium Controlled= 🧂 Vegetarian= 🥕

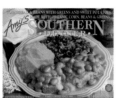

AMY'S
Southern Dinner
1 meal
310 Calories
🥕

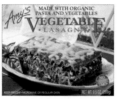

AMY'S
Vegetable Lasagna
1 container
310 Calories
🥕

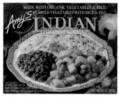

AMY'S
Indian Vegetable Korma
1 meal
310 Calories
🥕

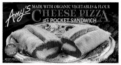

AMY'S
Cheese Pizza in a Pocket
Sandwich
1 sandwich
310 Calories
🧂 🥕

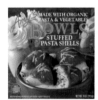

AMY'S
Stuffed Pasta Shells Bowl
1 package
310 Calories
🥕

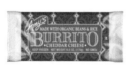

AMY'S
Cheddar Burrito
1 burrito
310 Calories
🥕

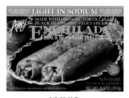

AMY'S
Light in Sodium Black
Bean Vegetable Enchilada
1 container
320 Calories
🧂 🥕

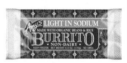

AMY'S
Light in Sodium Non Dairy
Beans & Rice Burrito
1 burrito
320 Calories
🧂 🥕

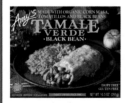

AMY'S
Black Bean Tamale Verde
1 meal
330 Calories
🥕

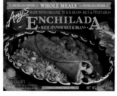

AMY'S
Whole Meals Black Bean
Enchilada
1 meal
330 Calories
🥕

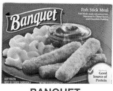

BANQUET
Fish Stick Meal
1 meal
310 Calories
🧂

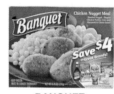

BANQUET
Chicken Nugget Meal
1 meal
320 Calories
🍞 🧂

ALL-AMERICAN DIET

90

Build-a-Meal
300-Calorie Lunch Entrées

Low Carb= 🍞 Sodium Controlled= 🧂 Vegetarian= 🌿

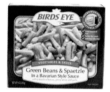

BIRDS EYE
Green Beans & Spaetzle
1 package
300 Calories
🌿

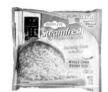

BIRDS EYE
Steamfresh Whole Grain
Brown Rice
1 bag
300 Calories
🧂 🌿

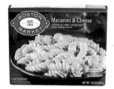

BOSTON MARKET
Macaroni and Cheese
1 meal
320 Calories
🌿

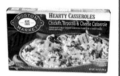

BOSTON MARKET
Chicken, Broccoli and
Cheese Casserole
1 meal
330 Calories

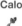

CAMPBELL'S
Cream of Asparagus
Condensed Soup
1 can
275 Calories
🍞 🌿

CAMPBELL'S
25% Less Sodium
Cream of Mushroom
Condensed Soup
1 can
275 Calories
🌿

CAMPBELL'S
Salisbury Steak with
Mushrooms & Onions
Chunky Soup
1 can
280 Calories

CAMPBELL'S
Grilled Chicken &
Sausage Gumbo
Chunky Soup
1 can
280 Calories

CAMPBELL'S
Grilled Chicken &
Sausage Gumbo Chunky
Soup Microwaveable
Bowl
1 bowl
280 Calories

CAMPBELL'S
Beef with White & Wild
Rice Chunky Soup
1 can
280 Calories

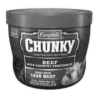

CAMPBELL'S
Beef with Country
Vegetables Chunky Soup
Microwaveable Bowl
1 bowl
300 Calories

CAMPBELL'S
Cream of Chicken with
Herbs Condensed Soup
1 can
300 Calories
🍞

Build-a-Meal
300-Calorie Lunch Entrées

Low Carb=🍞 Sodium Controlled=🧂 Vegetarian=🥕

CAMPBELL'S
Hearty Italian-Style
Wedding Chunky Soup
1 can
320 Calories

CAMPBELL'S
Creamy Tomato
Microwaveable Bowl
1 bowl
320 Calories
🥕

CAMPBELL'S
Select Harvest Italian
Sausage with Pasta &
Pepperoni Soup
1 can
320 Calories

CAMPBELL'S
Hearty Beef Barley
Chunky Soup
1 can
320 Calories

CAMPBELL'S
Lentil Condensed Soup
1 can
325 Calories

DR. PRAEGER'S
Minced Fish Sticks
9 fish sticks
330 Calories
🍞

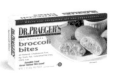

DR. PRAEGER'S
Broccoli Bites
6 pieces
330 Calories
🥕

HEALTHY CHOICE
Microwaveable Bowls
Minestrone
1 bowl
280 Calories
🧂

HEALTHY CHOICE
Microwaveable Bowls
Chicken Tortilla
1 bowl
280 Calories
🧂

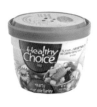

HEALTHY CHOICE
Microwaveable Bowls
Hearty Vegetable Barley
1 bowl
280 Calories
🧂 🥕

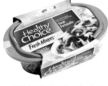

HEALTHY CHOICE
Fresh Mixers Steak
Portobello
1 package
290 Calories
🧂

HEALTHY CHOICE
Café Steamers Sweet
& Spicy Orange Zest
Chicken
1 meal
300 Calories
🧂

ALL-AMERICAN DIET

Build-a-Meal
300-Calorie Lunch Entrées

Low Carb= 🍞 **Sodium Controlled=** 🧂 **Vegetarian=** 🥕

HEALTHY CHOICE
Microwaveable Bowls
Traditional Lentil
1 bowl
300 Calories
🧂

HEALTHY CHOICE
Complete Meals Chicken
Pesto Alfredo
1 meal
300 Calories
🧂

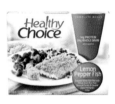

HEALTHY CHOICE
Complete Meals Lemon
Pepper Fish
1 meal
300 Calories
🧂

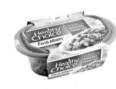

HEALTHY CHOICE
Fresh Mixers Rotini and
Zesty Marinara Sauce
1 package
300 Calories
🧂 🥕

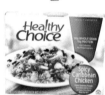

HEALTHY CHOICE
Select Entrées Spicy
Caribbean Chicken
1 meal
310 Calories

HEALTHY CHOICE
All Natural Three Cheese
Marinara
1 meal
310 Calories
🧂

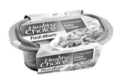

HEALTHY CHOICE
Fresh Mixers Chicken
Cacciatore
1 package
310 Calories
🧂

HEALTHY CHOICE
Café Steamers General
Tso's Spicy Chicken
1 meal
320 Calories

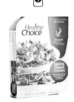

HEALTHY CHOICE
Steaming Entrées Sesame
Glazed Chicken
1 meal
320 Calories
🧂

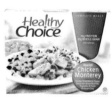

HEALTHY CHOICE
Complete Meals Roasted
Chicken Monterey
1 meal
320 Calories
🧂

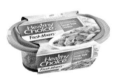

HEALTHY CHOICE
Fresh Mixers Tuscan Style
Chicken
1 package
320 Calories
🧂

HEALTHY CHOICE
Café Steamers Chicken
Margherita
1 meal
330 Calories
🧂

Build-a-Meal
300-Calorie Lunch Entrées

Low Carb= Sodium Controlled= Vegetarian=

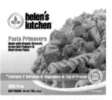

HELEN'S KITCHEN
Rotelli Primavera
1 container
330 Calories

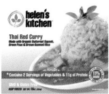

HELEN'S KITCHEN
Thai Red Curry
1 container
330 Calories

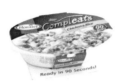

HORMEL
Compleats Chicken and Rice
1 package
280 Calories

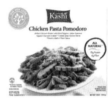

KASHI
Chicken Pasta Pomodoro
1 container
280 Calories

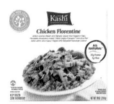

KASHI
Chicken Florentine
1 container
290 Calories

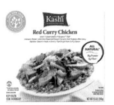

KASHI
Red Curry Chicken
1 container
300 Calories

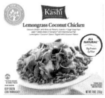

KASHI
Lemongrass Coconut Chicken
1 container
300 Calories

LEAN CUISINE
Market Creations Chicken Alfredo
1 meal
280 Calories

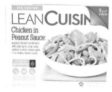

LEAN CUISINE
Spa Cuisine Chicken in Peanut Sauce
1 meal
280 Calories

LEAN CUISINE
Market Creations Mushroom Tortelloni
1 meal
280 Calories

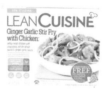

LEAN CUISINE
Spa Cuisine Ginger Garlic Stir Fry with Chicken
1 meal
280 Calories

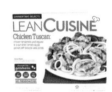

LEAN CUISINE
Dinnertime Selects Chicken Tuscan
1 meal
280 Calories

Build-a-Meal
300-Calorie Lunch Entrées

Low Carb= 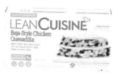 **Sodium Controlled=** **Vegetarian=**

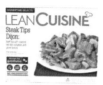

LEAN CUISINE
Dinnertime Selects Steak
Tips Dijon
1 meal
280 Calories

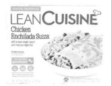

LEAN CUISINE
Simple Favorites Chicken
Enchilada Suiza
1 meal
280 Calories

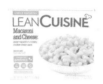

LEAN CUISINE
Simple Favorites Baja-
Style Chicken Quesadilla
1 quesadilla
280 Calories

LEAN CUISINE
Simple Favorites Macaroni
and Cheese
1 meal
290 Calories

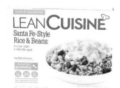

LEAN CUISINE
Simple Favorites Santa
Fe-Style Rice and Beans
1 meal
290 Calories

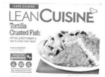

LEAN CUISINE
Cafe Cuisine Tortilla
Crusted Fish
1 meal
290 Calories

LEAN CUISINE
Cafe Cuisine Parmesan
Crusted Fish
1 meal
290 Calories

LEAN CUISINE
Market Creations Chicken
Poblano
1 meal
300 Calories

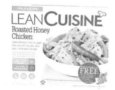

LEAN CUISINE
Spa Cuisine Roasted
Honey Chicken
1 meal
300 Calories

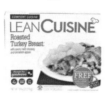

LEAN CUISINE
Comfort Cuisine Roasted
Turkey Breast
1 meal
300 Calories

LEAN CUISINE
Market Creations Chicken
Margherita
1 meal
300 Calories

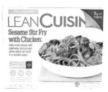

LEAN CUISINE
Spa Cuisine Sesame Stir
Fry with Chicken
1 meal
300 Calories

Build-a-Meal
300-Calorie Lunch Entrées

Low Carb= 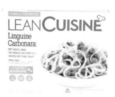 **Sodium Controlled=** **Vegetarian=**

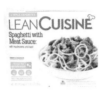

LEAN CUISINE
Simple Favorites
Spaghetti with Meat
Sauce
1 meal
300 Calories

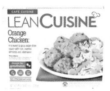

LEAN CUISINE
Cafe Cuisine Orange
Chicken
1 meal
300 Calories

LEAN CUISINE
Simple Favorites Linguine
Carbonara
1 meal
300 Calories

LEAN CUISINE
Comfort Cuisine
Chicken Parmesan
1 meal
310 Calories

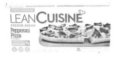

LEAN CUISINE
Simple Favorites
Pepperoni French Bread
Pizza
1 pizza
310 Calories

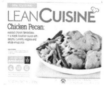

LEAN CUISINE
Spa Cuisine Chicken
Pecan
1 meal
310 Calories

LEAN CUISINE
Casual Cuisine
Mushroom Pizza
1 pizza
320 Calories

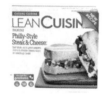

LEAN CUISINE
Casual Cuisine Philly-Style
Steak & Cheese Panini
1 panini
320 Calories

LEAN CUISINE
Casual Cuisine Southwest
Style Chicken Panini
1 panini
320 Calories

LEAN CUISINE
Spa Cuisine Apple
Cranberry Chicken
1 meal
320 Calories

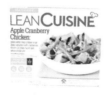

LEAN CUISINE
Casual Cuisine Bacon
Alfredo Pizza
1 pizza
320 Calories

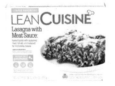

LEAN CUISINE
Simple Favorites Lasagna
with Meat Sauce
1 meal
320 Calories

ALL-AMERICAN DIET

Build-a-Meal
300-Calorie Lunch Entrées

Low Carb= **Sodium Controlled=** **Vegetarian=**

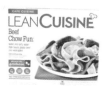

LEAN CUISINE
Cafe Cuisine Beef
Chow Fun
1 meal
320 Calories

LEAN CUISINE
Casual Cuisine Deep
Dish Roasted Vegetable
Pizza
1 pizza
320 Calories

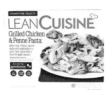

LEAN CUISINE
Dinnertime Selects Grilled
Chicken and Penne Pasta
1 meal
330 Calories

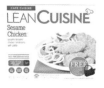

LEAN CUISINE
Cafe Cuisine Sesame
Chicken
1 meal
330 Calories

LEAN POCKETS
Pizzeria Sausage &
Pepperoni Pizza
1 piece
280 Calories

LEAN POCKETS
Meatballs & Mozzarella
1 piece
290 Calories

LEAN POCKETS
Pepperoni Pizza
1 piece
290 Calories

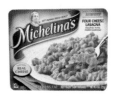

MICHELINA'S
Authentico Four
Cheese Lasagna
1 package
280 Calories

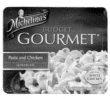

MICHELINA'S
Budget Gourmet Pasta
and Chicken in Cream
Sauce
1 package
280 Calories

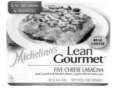

MICHELINA'S
Lean Gourmet Five
Cheese Lasagna
1 package
280 Calories

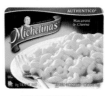

MICHELINA'S
Authentico Macaroni &
Cheese
1 package
300 Calories

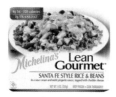

MICHELINA'S
Lean Gourmet Santa Fe
Style Rice & Beans
1 package
300 Calories

LUNCH ENTRÉES

97

Build-a-Meal
300-Calorie Lunch Entrées

Low Carb= Sodium Controlled= 🧂 Vegetarian= 🥕

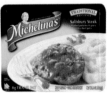

MICHELINA'S
Traditional Recipes
Salisbury Steak
1 package
330 Calories
🍞

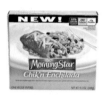

MORNINGSTAR FARMS
Chicken Enchilada
1 meal
280 Calories
🧂

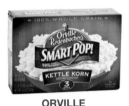

ORVILLE REDENBACHER'S
SmartPop! Kettle Korn
1 bag
280 Calories
🧂 🥕

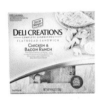

OSCAR MAYER
Deli Creations Flatbread
Sandwiches Chicken &
Bacon Ranch
1 package
320 Calories
🍞

OSCAR MAYER
Lunchables Turkey &
Cheddar with Crackers
1 package
330 Calories
🍞

READY PAC
Baby Spinach Complete
Salad
1 bag
280 Calories
🧂

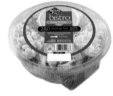

READY PAC
Santa Fe Style Caesar
Bistro Salad
1 package
280 Calories
🧂 🥕

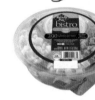

READY PAC
Cobb Bistro Salad
1 package
290 Calories
🧂

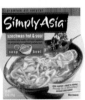

SIMPLY ASIA
Szechwan Hot & Sour
Soup Bowl
1 bowl
280 Calories
🥕

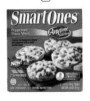

SMART ONES
Pepperoni Pizza Minis
Anytime Selections
4 pizzas
280 Calories
🥕

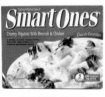

SMART ONES
Creamy Rigatoni with
Broccoli & Chicken
1 meal
280 Calories
🧂

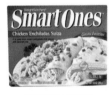

SMART ONES
Chicken Enchiladas Suiza
1 meal
290 Calories

Build-a-Meal
300-Calorie Lunch Entrées

Low Carb= **Sodium Controlled=** **Vegetarian=**

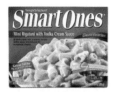

SMART ONES
Mini Rigatoni with Vodka
Cream Sauce
1 meal
290 Calories

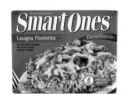

SMART ONES
Lasagna Florentine
1 meal
290 Calories

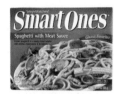

SMART ONES
Spaghetti with
Meat Sauce
1 meal
290 Calories

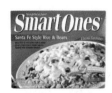

SMART ONES
Santa Fe Style Rice &
Beans
1 meal
310 Calories

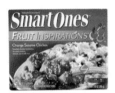

SMART ONES
Fruit Inspirations Orange
Sesame Chicken
1 meal
320 Calories

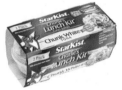

STARKIST
Charlie's Lunch Kit Tuna
Salad Chunk White
1 kit
290 calories

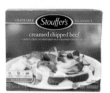

STOUFFER'S
Craveable Classics
Creamed Chipped Beef
1 meal
280 Calories

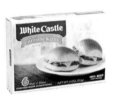

WHITE CASTLE
Microwaveable Cheese-
burgers
2 burgers
310 Calories

Build-a-Meal
350-Calorie Lunch Entrées

Low Carb= 🍞 **Sodium Controlled=** 🧂 **Vegetarian=** 🌿

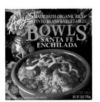

AMY'S
Santa Fe Enchilada Bowl
1 bowl
350 Calories
🌿

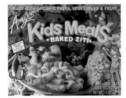

AMY'S
Baked Ziti Kids Meal
1 meal
360 Calories
🧂 🌿

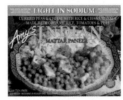

AMY'S
Non-Dairy Vegetable
Pot Pie
1 pie
360 Calories
🌿

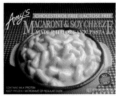

AMY'S
Light in Sodium Indian
Mattar Paneer
1 meal
370 Calories
🧂 🌿

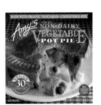

AMY'S
Macaroni & Soy Cheeze
1 container
370 Calories
🧂 🌿

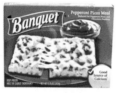

BANQUET
Pepperoni Pizza Meal
1 meal
340 Calories

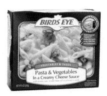

BIRDS EYE
Pasta & Vegetables in a
Creamy Cheese Sauce
1 package
340 Calories
🌿

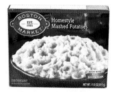

BOSTON MARKET
Homestyle Mashed
Potatoes
1 package
340 Calories
🌿

CAMPBELL'S
Original SpaghettiOs
1 can
340 Calories
🌿

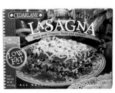

CEDARLANE
Low Fat Garden Veg-
etable Lasagna
1 package
360 Calories
🌿

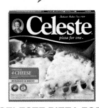

**CELESTE PIZZA FOR
ONE**
Four Cheese
1 pizza
350 Calories
🌿

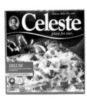

CELESTE
Pizza for One Deluxe
1 pizza
370 Calories

ALL-AMERICAN DIET

Build-a-Meal
350-Calorie Lunch Entrées

Low Carb= **Sodium Controlled=** **Vegetarian=**

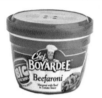

CHEF BOYARDEE
Beefaroni Microwaveable
Big Size Bowl
1 14.5-ounce bowl
368 Calories

FRESH EXPRESS
Caesar Kit
1 package
360 Calories

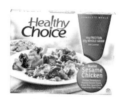

HEALTHY CHOICE
Complete Meals Roasted
Sesame Chicken
1 meal
340 Calories

HEALTHY CHOICE
All Natural Asian
Potstickers
1 meal
340 Calories

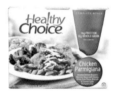

HEALTHY CHOICE
Complete Meals Chicken
Parmigiana
1 meal
350 Calories

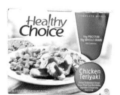

HEALTHY CHOICE
Complete Meals Chicken
Teriyaki
1 meal
350 Calories

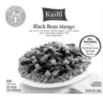

KASHI
Black Bean Mango
1 container
340 Calories

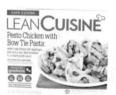

LEAN CUISINE
Cafe Cuisine Pesto
Chicken with Bow
Tie Pasta
1 meal
340 Calories

LEAN CUISINE
Simple Favorites Deluxe
French Bread Pizza
1 pizza
340 Calories

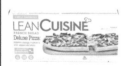

LEAN CUISINE
Casual Cuisine BBQ-
Recipe Chicken Pizza,
Wood Fire Style
1 pizza
340 Calories

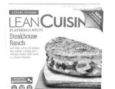

LEAN CUISINE
Casual Cuisine
Steakhouse Ranch
Flatbread Melt
1 melt
350 Calories

LEAN CUISINE
Casual Cuisine Chicken
Philly Flatbread Melt
1 melt
350 Calories

Build-a-Meal
350-Calorie Lunch Entrées

Low Carb= **Sodium Controlled=** **Vegetarian=**

LEAN CUISINE
Casual Cuisine Roasted
Garlic Chicken Pizza
Wood Fired
1 pizza
350 Calories

LEAN CUISINE
Casual Cuisine Sun Dried
Tomato Basil Chicken
Flatbread Melt
1 meal
360 Calories

LEAN CUISINE
Casual Cuisine Chicken
Club Panini
1 panini
360 Calories

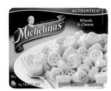

MICHELINA'S
Authentico Wheels &
Cheese
1 package
350 Calories

OSCAR MAYER
Deli Creations Cracker
Combinations Turkey
& Chicken with Swiss
& Cheddar
1 package
340 Calories

OSCAR MAYER
Lunchables Ham & Ched-
dar with Crackers
1 package
340 Calories

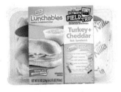

OSCAR MAYER
Lunchables Turkey &
Cheddar Sub Sandwich
1 package
370 Calories

PROGRESSO
Traditional New England
Clam Chowder
1 can
360 Calories

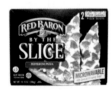

RED BARON
Pepperoni Pizza By
the Slice
1 slice
360 Calories

SABRA
Hummus with Pretzels
Roasted Red Pepper
1 package
370 Calories

STOUFFER'S
Farmers' Harvest Grilled
Chicken Fettuccini Alfredo
1 meal
350 Calories

Build-a-Meal
400-Calorie Lunch Entrées

Low Carb= Sodium Controlled= 🧂 Vegetarian= 🥕

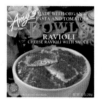

AMY'S
Cheese Ravioli Bowl
1 bowl
380 Calories
🥕

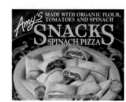

AMY'S
Spinach Pizza Snacks
1 box
380 Calories
🥕

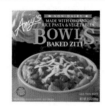

AMY'S
Non-Dairy Baked Ziti Bowl
1 bowl
390 Calories
🧂 🥕

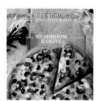

AMY'S
Mushroom & Olive Pizza
½ pizza
390 Calories
🥕

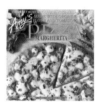

AMY'S
Single Serve Margherita
Pizza
1 pizza
400 Calories
🥕

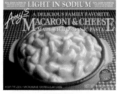

AMY'S
Light in Sodium Macaroni
and Cheese
1 container
400 Calories
🧂 🥕

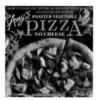

AMY'S
Roasted Vegetable Pizza
½ pizza
420 Calories
🥕

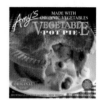

AMY'S
Vegetable Pot Pie
1 pie
420 Calories
🧂 🥕

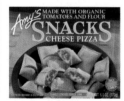

AMY'S
Cheese Pizza Snacks
1 box
420 Calories
🥕

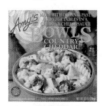

AMY'S
Country Cheddar Bowl
1 bowl
430 Calories
🥕

AMY'S
Light in Sodium Country
Cheddar Bowl
1 bowl
430 Calories
🧂 🥕

ANNIE CHUN'S
Thai Peanut Noodle
Express
1 container
400 Calories
🥕

Build-a-Meal
400-Calorie Lunch Entrées

Low Carb= 🍞 **Sodium Controlled=** 🧂 **Vegetarian=** 🥕

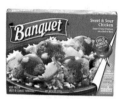

BANQUET
Sweet and Sour Chicken
1 meal
390 Calories
🧂

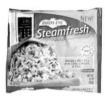
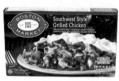

BIRDS EYE
Steamfresh Brown & Wild
Rice with Corn,
Carrots & Peas
1 bag
380 Calories
🧂 🥕

BOSTON MARKET
Southwest Style Grilled
Chicken Meal
1 meal
410 Calories

CAMPBELL'S
Baked Potato with Ched-
dar & Bacon Bits Chunky
Soup
1 can
380 Calories

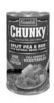

CAMPBELL'S
Split Pea and Ham
Chunky Soup
1 can
380 Calories

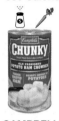

CAMPBELL'S
Old Fashioned Potato
Ham Chowder Chunky
Soup
1 can
380 Calories

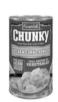

CAMPBELL'S
Chicken Corn Chowder
Chunky Soup
1 can
400 Calories

CAMPBELL'S
New England Clam
Chowder Chunky Soup
Microwaveable Bowl
1 bowl
400 Calories

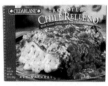

CEDARLANE
Roasted Chile Relleno
1 package
400 Calories

CELESTE
Pizza for One Pepperoni
1 pizza
410 Calories

CHEF BOYARDEE
Mini Ravioli Microwave-
able Big Size Bowl
1 14.25-ounce bowl
384 Calories

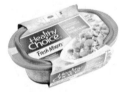

HEALTHY CHOICE
Fresh Mixers Sesame
Teriyaki Chicken
1 package
380 Calories

Build-a-Meal
400-Calorie Lunch Entrées

Low Carb= Sodium Controlled= Vegetarian= 🌿

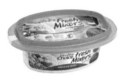

HEALTHY CHOICE
Fresh Mixers Sweet and
Sour Chicken
1 package
390 Calories

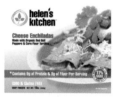

HELEN'S KITCHEN
Cheese Enchiladas
1 container
420 Calories
🌿

HORMEL
Microwaveable Bowls
Chili, No Beans
1 bowl
380 Calories

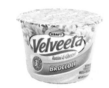

KRAFT
Velveeta Rotini & Cheese
with Broccoli
1 container
380 Calories
🌿

LEAN CUISINE
Casual Cuisine Pepperoni
Pizza
1 container
380 Calories

LEAN CUISINE
Casual Cuisine Deep Dish
Three Meat Pizza
1 container
390 Calories

NATURE'S PATH
Organic Frosted Toaster
Pastries, Wildberry Acai
2 pastries
420 Calories
🧂 🌿

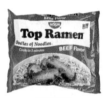

NISSIN
Top Ramen, Beef Flavor
1 package
380 Calories

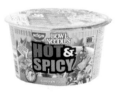

NISSIN
Bowl Noodles Hot &
Spicy Chicken Flavor
1 container
420 Calories

OREIDA
Bagel Bites, Three
Cheese
9 pieces
428 Calories
🌿

ORGANIC BISTRO
Alaskan Salmon Cake
1 meal
410 Calories
🧂

OSCAR MAYER
Deli Creations Steakhouse
Cheddar
1 package
430 Calories

Build-a-Meal
400-Calorie Lunch Entrées

Low Carb=  **Sodium Controlled=** 🧂 **Vegetarian=** 🌿

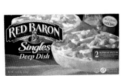

RED BARON
Singles Deep Dish
Supreme Pizzas
1 pizza
420 Calories

SABRA
Hummus with Pretzels,
Classic
1 package
380 Calories
🌿

SMART ONES
Artisan Creations Four
Cheese Pizza
1 meal
380 Calories
🌿

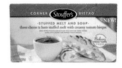

STOUFFER'S
Corner Bistro Stuffed Melt
& Soup Three Cheese &
Ham Melt with Creamy
Tomato Soup
1 meal
380 Calories

STOUFFER'S
Corner Bistro Flatbread
Melt Steak Mushroom
Cheddar
1 sandwich
390 Calories

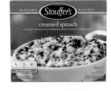

STOUFFER'S
Craveable Recipes
Creamed Spinach
1 meal
400 Calories
🌿

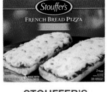

STOUFFER'S
Extra Cheese French
Bread Pizza
1 piece
400 Calories
🌿

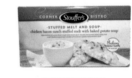

STOUFFER'S
Corner Bistro Stuffed Melt
& Soup Chicken Bacon
Ranch with Baked Potato
Soup
1 meal
430 Calories

STOUFFER'S
Corner Bistro Stromboli
Pepperoni & Provolone
1 stromboli
430 Calories

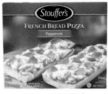

STOUFFER'S
Pepperoni French Bread
Pizza
1 piece
430 Calories

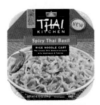

THAI KITCHEN
Spicy Thai Basil Rice
Noodle Cart
1 package
430 Calories
🌿

UNCLE BEN'S
Ready Whole Grain
Medley Chicken Medley
1 package
420 Calories

ALL-AMERICAN DIET

Build-a-Meal 50-Calorie
Lunch Sides and Afternoon Snacks

Low Carb= Sodium Controlled= Vegetarian=

AMY'S
Fat Free Chunky Vegetable Soup
½ can
60 Calories

ANNIE'S
Organic Bunny Fruit Snacks, Tropical Treat
1 pouch
70 Calories

ANNIE'S
Organic Bunny Fruit Snacks, Berry Patch
1 pouch
70 Calories

CAMPBELL'S
Chicken & Stars Soup at Hand
1 container
70 Calories

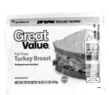

GREAT VALUE
Fat Free Turkey Breast
2 slices
40 Calories

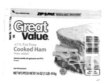

GREAT VALUE
97% Fat Free Cooked Ham
2 slices
60 Calories

HILLSHIRE FARM
Deli Select Honey Roasted Turkey Breast
6 slices
60 Calories

KRAFT
Polly-O Twists, Mozzarella and Cheddar
1 stick
60 Calories

KRAFT
Singles, American
1 slice
70 Calories

KRAFT
Polly-O String Cheese, Mozzarella
1 stick
70 Calories

THE LAUGHING COW
Light Queso Fresco & Chipotle
1 wedge
35 Calories

THE LAUGHING COW
Light Blue Cheese
1 wedge
35 Calories

Build-a-Meal 50-Calorie
Lunch Sides and Afternoon Snacks

Low Carb= **Sodium Controlled=** 🧂 **Vegetarian=** 🥕

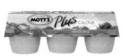

MOTT'S
Plus Calcium Harvest
Apple Sauce
1 container
50 Calories

🧂 🥕

ORGANIC VALLEY
Provolone Cheese
1 slice
70 Calories

🥪 🧂 🥕

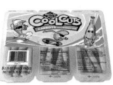

**READY PAC COOL
CUTS**
Carrots with Ranch Dip
Snack Pac
1 package
70 Calories

🥪 🧂 🥕

SARGENTO
Light String Cheese
1 stick
50 Calories

🥪 🧂 🥕

SARGENTO
Reduced Fat Colby-Jack
Cheese Sticks
1 stick
60 Calories

🥪 🧂 🥕

SARGENTO
Reduced Fat Colby-Jack
Sliced Cheese
1 slice
60 Calories

🥪 🧂 🥕

SARGENTO
Reduced Fat Pepper Jack
Sliced Cheese
1 slice
60 Calories

🥪 🧂 🥕

SARGENTO
Reduced Fat Swiss Deli
Style Sliced Cheese
1 slice
60 Calories

🥪 🧂 🥕

SARGENTO
Natural Baby Swiss Deli
Style Sliced Cheese
1 slice
70 Calories

🥪 🧂 🥕

SARGENTO
String Cheese
1 stick
70 Calories

🥪 🧂 🥕

**STRETCH ISLAND
FRUIT CO.**
All-Natural Fruit Strip,
Ripened Raspberry
1 strip
45 Calories

🧂 🥕

**STRETCH ISLAND
FRUIT CO.**
All-Natural Fruit Strip,
Orchard Cherry
1 strip
45 Calories

🧂 🥕

Build-a-Meal 100-Calorie
Lunch Sides and Afternoon Snacks

Low Carb= Sodium Controlled= Vegetarian=

ALEXIA
Whole Grain Rolls
1 roll
100 Calories

ALEXIA
Ciabatta Rolls
1 roll
100 Calories

AMY'S
Low Fat Minestrone Soup
½ can
90 Calories

AMY'S
Light in Sodium Low Fat
Minestrone Soup
½ can
90 Calories

AMY'S
Low Fat Split Pea Soup
½ can
100 Calories

AMY'S
Low Fat No Chicken
Noodle Soup
½ can
100 Calories

AMY'S
Light in Sodium Low Fat
Cream of Tomato Soup
½ can
110 Calories

AMY'S
Chunky Tomato Bisque
Soup
½ can
130 Calories

AMY'S
Light in Sodium Chunky
Tomato Bisque Soup
½ can
130 Calories

ARNOLD'S
Sandwich Thins Multi
Grain
1 thin
100 Calories

CAMPBELL'S
Select Harvest Light
Italian-Style Vegetable
Soup
1 can
100 Calories

CAMPBELL'S
Select Harvest Light
Southwestern-Style
Vegetable Soup
1 can
100 Calories
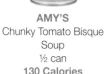

LUNCH SIDES AND AFTERNOON SNACKS

Build-a-Meal 100-Calorie
Lunch Sides and Afternoon Snacks

Low Carb= 🍞 **Sodium Controlled=** 🧂 **Vegetarian=** 🍴

CAMPBELL'S
Select Harvest Light
Italian-Style Vegetable
Microwaveable Bowl
1 bowl
100 Calories
🍴

CAMPBELL'S
Hearty Chicken with
Vegetables Chunky Soup
½ **can**
110 Calories

CAMPBELL'S
Savory Pot Roast Chunky
Soup
½ can
120 Calories

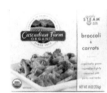

CASCADIAN FARM
Broccoli and Carrots
1 box
102 Calories
🍴

CASCADIAN FARM
Harvest Berry Chewy
Granola Bars
1 bar
130 Calories
🧂 🍴

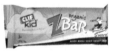

CLIF KID
ZBar S'mores
1 bar
130 Calories
🧂 🍴

DANNON
Light & Fit Blackberry
1 container
80 Calories
🧂 🍴

DEL MONTE
100 Calorie Fruit Cocktail
1 can
100 Calories
🧂 🍴

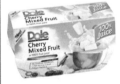

DOLE
Cherry Mixed Fruit
1 container
70 Calories
🧂 🍴

DOLE
Real Fruit Bites with
Yogurt and Whole Grain
Oats Apple Chunks
1 pouch
80 Calories
🧂 🍴

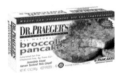

DR. PRAEGER'S
Broccoli Pancakes
1 pancake
80 Calories
🧂 🍴

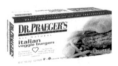

DR. PRAEGER'S
Italian Veggie Burgers
1 burger
110 Calories
🧂 🍴

Build-a-Meal 100-Calorie
Lunch Sides and Afternoon Snacks

Low Carb= **Sodium Controlled=** **Vegetarian=**

EMERALD
100 Calorie Packs Natural
Walnuts and Almonds
1 pouch
100 Calories

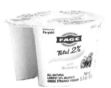

FAGE
Total 2% with Blueberry
Greek Yogurt
1 container
130 Calories

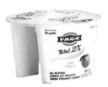

FAGE
Total 2% with Peach
Greek Yogurt
1 container
130 Calories

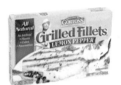

GORTON'S
Grilled Lemon Pepper
Fish Fillets
1 fillet
100 Calories

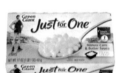

GREEN GIANT
Just for One Niblets Corn
in Butter Sauce
1 container
80 Calories

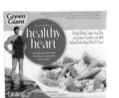

GREEN GIANT
Healthy Heart
1 box
83 Calories

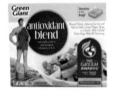

GREEN GIANT
Antioxidant Blend
1 box
100 Calories

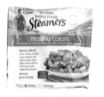

GREEN GIANT
Steamers Healthy Colors
Market Blend
1 package
100 Calories

HORMEL
Hard Salami
6 slices
110 Calories

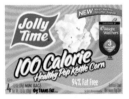

JOLLY TIME
100 Calorie Healthy Pop
Kettle Corn
1 bag
90 Calories

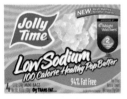

JOLLY TIME
Low Sodium 100 Calorie
Healthy Pop Butter
1 bag
90 Calories

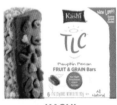

KASHI
TLC Fruit & Grain Bars,
Pumpkin Pecan
1 bar
120 Calories

LUNCH SIDES AND AFTERNOON SNACKS

Build-a-Meal 100-Calorie Lunch Sides and Afternoon Snacks

Low Carb= **Sodium Controlled=** **Vegetarian=**

KEEBLER
100 Calorie Right Bites Variety Pack (Fudge Grahams, Cheez-It, Mini Fudge Stripes)
100 Calories

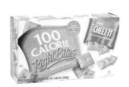

KELLOGG'S
100 Calorie Right Bites Cheez-It
1 pouch
100 Calories

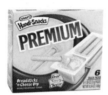

KRAFT
Handi-Snacks Premium Breadsticks 'n Cheese Dip
1 package
110 Calories

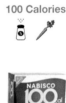

KUDOS
100 Calorie Bars
1 bar
100 Calories

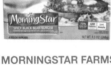

MORNINGSTAR FARMS
Spicy Black Bean Burger
1 patty
120 Calories

MOTT'S
Cinnamon Apple Sauce
1 4-ounce container
100 Calories

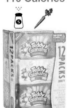

NABISCO
Teddy Grahams Variety Pack
1 pouch
90 Calories

NABISCO
100 Cal Sweet & Salty
1 pouch
100 Calories

NABISCO
Ritz Crackerfuls Cheddar Cheese & Bacon
1 package
130 Calories

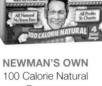

NATURE VALLEY
Granola Thins Crispy Squares
1 pouch
90 Calories

NEWMAN'S OWN
100 Calorie Natural Popcorn
1 mini bag
100 Calories

ORGANIC VALLEY
Baby Swiss Cheese
1 slice
80 Calories

ALL-AMERICAN DIET

Build-a-Meal 100-Calorie
Lunch Sides and Afternoon Snacks

Low Carb= **Sodium Controlled=** 🧂 **Vegetarian=** 🥕

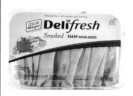

OSCAR MAYER
Deli Fresh Smoked Ham
½ 9-ounce package
113 Calories

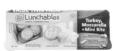

OSCAR MAYER
Lunchables Turkey, Moz-
zarella & Mini Ritz
1 package
130 Calories

PEPPERIDGE FARM
100 Calorie Pouches
Goldfish Flavor Blasted
Xtra Cheddar
1 pouch
100 Calories

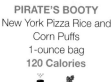

PIRATE'S BOOTY
New York Pizza Rice and
Corn Puffs
1-ounce bag
120 Calories

PIRATE'S BOOTY
Aged White Cheddar Rice
and Corn Puffs
1-ounce bag
130 Calories

PIRATE'S BOOTY
Veggie Rice and Corn
Puffs
1-ounce bag
130 Calories

POP CHIPS
Original Potato
1 0.8-ounce bag
100 Calories

POP CHIPS
Sour Cream & Onion
Potato
1 0.8-ounce bag
100 Calories

POP CHIPS
Barbeque Potato
1 0.8-ounce bag
100 Calories

POP CHIPS
Parmesan Garlic Potato
1 0.8-ounce bag
100 Calories

PRINGLES
Baked Wheat Stix,
Jalapeño
1 package
90 Calories

PRINGLES
Baked Wheat Stix, Pizza
1 package
90 Calories

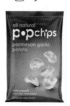

LUNCH SIDES AND AFTERNOON SNACKS

Build-a-Meal 100-Calorie
Lunch Sides and Afternoon Snacks

Low Carb= 🍞 **Sodium Controlled=** 🧂 **Vegetarian=** 🥕

PRINGLES
100 Calorie Pack Original
1 tub
100 Calories
🧂 🥕

SARGENTO
Colby-Jack Cheese Sticks
1 piece
80 Calories
🍞 🧂 🥕

SARGENTO
MooTown Cheese Dip
& Pretzel Sticks
1 package
80 Calories
🧂 🥕

SARGENTO
Mild Cheddar Snack Bars
1 piece
90 Calories
🍞 🧂 🥕

SARGENTO
MooTown Cheese Dip
& Cracker Sticks
1 package
100 Calories
🧂 🥕

SARGENTO
Cheddar Cheese Sticks
1 stick
100 Calories
🍞 🧂 🥕

SARGENTO
Colby-Jack Cheese
Cubes
7 cubes
110 Calories
🍞 🧂 🥕

**SNYDER'S OF
HANOVER**
100 Calorie Pack Pretzel
Snaps
1 1-ounce bag
100 Calories
🧂

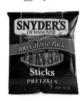

**SNYDER'S OF
HANOVER**
100 Calorie Pack Pretzel
Sticks
1 1-ounce bag
100 Calories
🧂

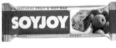

SOYJOY
All Natural Fruit & Soy Bar
Berry
1 bar
130 Calories
🥕

STONYFIELD
0% Fat Strawberry Fruit
on the Bottom
1 container
110 Calories
🧂 🥕

STONYFIELD
Low Fat Mango Honey
Smooth and Creamy
1 container
130 Calories
🧂 🥕

Build-a-Meal 100-Calorie
Lunch Sides and Afternoon Snacks

Low Carb= Sodium Controlled=  Vegetarian=

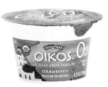

STONYFIELD
Oikos Greek Yogurt,
Strawberry
1 container
110 Calories

STONYFIELD
0% Fat Lemon Smooth
and Creamy
1 container
130 Calories

SUN-MAID
Vanilla Yogurt Raisins
1 1-ounce box
120 Calories

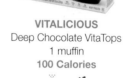

VITALICIOUS
Deep Chocolate VitaTops
1 muffin
100 Calories

WEIGHT WATCHERS
Pita Pockets
1 piece
100 Calories

WHOLLY GUACAMOLE
100 Cal Snack Packs
1 pouch
100 Calories

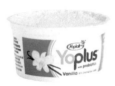

YOPLAIT
Light Fat Free Harvest
Peach
1 container
100 Calories

YOPLAIT
Yo Plus Vanilla
1 container
110 Calorie

Build-a-Meal 150-Calorie
Lunch Sides and Afternoon Snacks

Low Carb= **Sodium Controlled=** **Vegetarian=**

AMY'S
Low Fat Black Bean
Vegetable Soup
½ can
140 Calories

AMY'S
Rustic Italian Vegetable
Soup
½ can
140 Calories

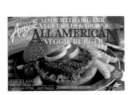

AMY'S
All American Veggie
Burger
1 burger
140 Calories

AMY'S
Hearty Spanish Rice and
Red Bean Soup
½ can
140 Calories

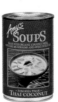

AMY'S
Tom Ka Phak Thai
Coconut Soup
½ can
140 Calories

AMY'S
Semi-Condensed Cream
of Mushroom Soup
½ can
150 Calories

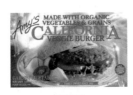

AMY'S
California Veggie Burger
1 burger
150 Calories

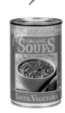

AMY'S
Light in Sodium Lentil
Vegetable Soup
½ can
160 Calories

AMY'S
Light in Sodium
Shepherd's Pie
1 pie
160 Calories

AMY'S
Lentil Vegetable Soup
½ can
160 Calories

BREAKSTONE'S
100 Calorie Cottage
Doubles, Apples
& Cinnamon
1 container
140 Calories

BUMBLE BEE
Fat Free Tuna Salad with
Crackers
1 package
150 Calories

ALL-AMERICAN DIET

Build-a-Meal 150-Calorie
Lunch Sides and Afternoon Snacks

Low Carb= Sodium Controlled= Vegetarian=

BUMBLE BEE
Prime Fillet Pink Salmon
Steak, Lemon & Dill
1 package
150 Calories

CAMPBELL'S
98% Fat Free Cream of
Celery Condensed Soup
1 can
150 Calories

CAMPBELL'S
Healthy Request Home-
style Chicken Noodle
Condensed Soup
1 can
150 Calories

CAMPBELL'S
Select Harvest Light
Maryland-Style Crab
Soup
1 can
160 Calories

DIET DETECTIVE'S WHAT YOU NEED TO KNOW

SOUP SMART

Ahhh, a good hot bowl of soup—not to sound like a commercial, but it brings back fond memories. Soup is great if you're looking for something to fill you up. Because soups are water based, they tend to fill you up and make you feel less hungry without adding too many calories, so you eat less as a result—which is certainly very helpful in terms of losing weight. Barbara Rolls, PhD, a professor of nutrition at Pennsylvania State University, has led several studies that show that eating soup can help you lose weight. One study actually found that eating soup before your meal could reduce your mealtime consumption by as much as 100 calories. Try to include soup in your Build-a-Meal plan at least once a day. Some of the sample plans I've provided include soup as a side for both lunch and dinner. Soup helps! Also, if your plan calls for half a can, simply put the remaining soup in a covered plastic storage container and stick it in the fridge to use another day.

Build-a-Meal 150-Calorie Lunch Sides and Afternoon Snacks

Low Carb= **Sodium Controlled=** **Vegetarian=**

CAMPBELL'S
25% Less Sodium
Chicken Noodle
Condensed Soup
1 can
150 Calories

CAMPBELL'S
Chicken Won Ton
Condensed Soup
1 can
150 Calories

CAMPBELL'S
Select Harvest Garden
Recipes Vegetable
Medley Soup
1 can
160 Calories

CAMPBELL'S
Healthy Kids Chicken
Alphabet Condensed
Soup
1 can
161 Calories

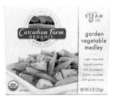

CASCADIAN FARM
Garden Vegetable Medley
1 box
138 Calories

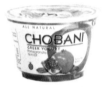

CHOBANI
Nonfat Greek Yogurt,
Pomegranate
1 container
140 Calories

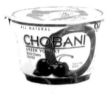

CHOBANI
Nonfat Greek Yogurt,
Black Cherry
1 container
150 Calories

DOLE
Fruit Crisps,
Pineapple Mango
1 container
150 Calories

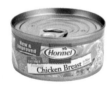

HORMEL
Premium Canned Chicken
Breast in Water
1 can
150 Calories

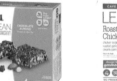

KASHI
GoLean Crunchy! Protein
& Fiber Bars, Chocolate
Almond
1 bar
170 Calories

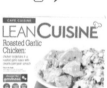

LEAN CUISINE
Cafe Cuisine Roasted
Garlic Chicken
1 meal
170 Calories

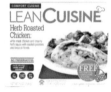

LEAN CUISINE
Comfort Cuisine Herb
Roasted Chicken
1 meal
170 Calories

Build-a-Meal 150-Calorie
Lunch Sides and Afternoon Snacks

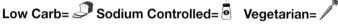

Low Carb= Sodium Controlled= Vegetarian=

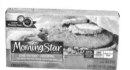

MORNINGSTAR FARMS
Chik Patties Original
1 patty
140 Calories

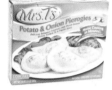

MRS. T'S
Potato & Onion Pierogies
3 pieces
160 Calories

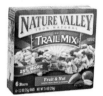

NATURE VALLEY
Chewy Trail Mix Fruit &
Nut Bars
1 bar
140 Calories

NATURE'S PATH
Organic Chewy Granola
Bars, Peanut Buddy
1 bar
140 Calories

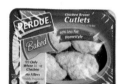

PERDUE
Baked Chicken Breast
Cutlets, Homestyle
1 cutlet
160 Calories

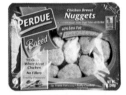

PERDUE
Baked Chicken Breast
Nuggets, Whole Grain
Breaded
4 nuggets
170 Calories

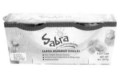

SABRA
Hummus Singles
1 2-ounce container
140 Calories

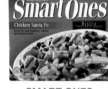

SMART ONES
Chicken Santa Fe
1 meal
140 Calories

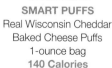

SMART PUFFS
Real Wisconsin Cheddar
Baked Cheese Puffs
1-ounce bag
140 Calories

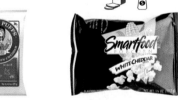

SMARTFOOD
White Cheddar Popcorn
1 1-ounce bag
160 Calories

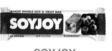

SOYJOY
Baked Whole Soy & Fruit
Bar, Blueberry
1 bar
140 Calories

YOPLAIT
Whips Strawberry Mist
1 container
140 Calories

Build-a-Meal 200-Calorie Lunch Sides and Afternoon Snacks

Low Carb= 🍞 **Sodium Controlled=** 🧂 **Vegetarian=** 🥕

AMY'S
Lentil Soup
½ can
180 Calories
🥕

AMY'S
Hearty French Country
Vegetable Soup
½ can
180 Calories
🥕

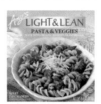

AMY'S
Light & Lean Pasta &
Veggies
1 container
210 Calories
🧂 🥕

AMY'S
Low Fat Medium Black
Bean Chili
½ can
200 Calories
🥕

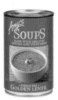

AMY'S
Indian Dal Golden Lentil
Soup
½ can
220 Calories
🥕

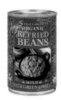

AMY'S
Refried Beans, Mild with
Green Chiles
½ can
228 Calories
🥕

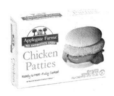

APPLEGATE FARMS
Chicken Patties
1 patty
180 Calories
🍞 🧂

CAMPBELL'S
Beef Noodle Condensed
Soup
1 can
175 Calories

CAMPBELL'S
Healthy Request Chicken
Noodle Condensed Soup
1 can
175 Calories

CAMPBELL'S
98% Fat Free Cream of
Chicken Condensed Soup
1 can
175 Calories

CAMPBELL'S
French Onion
Condensed Soup
1 can
175 Calories
🍞

CAMPBELL'S
Manhattan Clam Chowder
Condensed Soup
1 can
175 Calories

Build-a-Meal 200-Calorie
Lunch Sides and Afternoon Snacks

Low Carb= Sodium Controlled= 🧂 Vegetarian= 🌿

CAMPBELL'S
Select Harvest Roasted
Chicken with Rotini &
Penne Pasta Soup
1 can
180 Calories

CAMPBELL'S
Grilled Chicken with Veg-
etables & Pasta Chunky
Soup
1 can
200 Calories

CAMPBELL'S
Select Harvest Garden
Recipes Harvest Tomato
with Basil Soup
1 can
200 Calories
🌿

CAMPBELL'S
Golden Mushroom
Condensed Soup
1 can
200 Calories

CAMPBELL'S
Old Fashioned Vegetable
Beef Chunky Soup
Microwaveable Bowl
1 bowl
200 Calories

CAMPBELL'S
Healthy Kids Chicken
Noodle O's Condensed
Soup
1 can
207 Calories

CAMPBELL'S
Healthy Kids Mega
Noodle Condensed Soup
1 can
207 Calories

CAMPBELL'S
Savory Vegetable Chunky
Soup
1 can
220 Calories

CAMPBELL'S
Select Harvest Mexican-
Style Chicken Tortilla
Soup
1 can
220 Calories

CAMPBELL'S
Savory Chicken with
White & Wild Rice Chunky
Soup
1 can
220 Calories

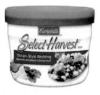

CAMPBELL'S
Select Harvest Italian-
Style Wedding Micro-
waveable Bowl
1 bowl
220 Calories

CAMPBELL'S
Cream of Potato
Condensed Soup
1 can
225 Calories
🌿

Build-a-Meal 200-Calorie
Lunch Sides and Afternoon Snacks

Low Carb= 🍞 **Sodium Controlled=** 🧂 **Vegetarian=** 🍴

CAMPBELL'S
Tomato Condensed Soup
1 can
225 Calories
🍴

CAMPBELL'S
Cream of Celery
Condensed Soup
1 can
225 Calories
🍴

CAMPBELL'S
New England Clam
Chowder Condensed
Soup
1 can
225 Calories

CHEF BOYARDEE
Rice with Chicken and
Vegetables Microwave-
able Bowl
1 7.25-ounce bowl
230 Calories

CLIF
Mojo Bar, Peanut Butter
Pretzel
1 bar
190 Calories
🧂 🍴

CLIF
Mojo Bar, Mountain Mix
1 bar
190 Calories
🧂 🍴

EARTH'S BEST
Whole Grain Cheese
Pizza
1 pizza
190 Calories
🧂 🍴

FRESH EXPRESS
Chicken Caesar Gourmet
Café Salad
1 container
180 Calories
🍞

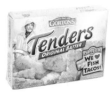

GORTON'S
Tenders Original Batter
Whole Fish Fillets
3 pieces
230 Calories

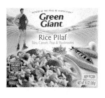

GREEN GIANT
Rice Pilaf
1 box
200 Calories
🍴

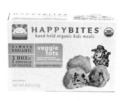

HAPPYBITES
Veggie Tots
8 pieces
220 Calories
🧂 🍴

HEALTHY CHOICE
Microwaveable Bowls
Chicken Noodle
1 bowl
180 Calories

Build-a-Meal 200-Calorie
Lunch Sides and Afternoon Snacks

Low Carb= 🍞 **Sodium Controlled=** 🧂 **Vegetarian=** 🌿

HEALTHY CHOICE
Microwaveable Bowls
Country Vegetable
1 bowl
180 Calories

HEALTHY CHOICE
Canned Soup, Tomato
Basil
1 can
200 Calories

HEALTHY CHOICE
Microwaveable Bowls
Chicken with Rice
1 bowl
200 Calories

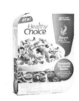

HEALTHY CHOICE
Steaming Entrées Porta-
bella Parmesan Risotto
1 meal
220 Calories
🧂🌿

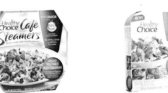

HEALTHY CHOICE
Café Steamers Vegetable
Mediterranean
1 meal
220 Calories
🧂🌿

HEALTHY CHOICE
Steaming Entrées Chicken
Romana Fresca
1 meal
230 Calories
🧂

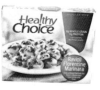

HEALTHY CHOICE
Select Entrées Ravioli
Florentine Marinara
1 meal
230 Calories
🧂🌿

HORMEL
Turkey Chili with Beans
½ can
210 Calories

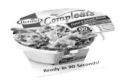

HORMEL
Compleats Cheese and
Spinach Ravioli
1 package
230 Calories
🌿

JOSÉ OLÉ
Taquitos, Chicken
3 taquitos
200 Calories
🧂

JOSÉ OLÉ
Taquitos, Shredded Steak
3 taquitos
210 Calories
🧂

JOSÉ OLÉ
Taquitos, Chicken and
Cheese
2 taquitos
230 Calories

Build-a-Meal 200-Calorie
Lunch Sides and Afternoon Snacks

Low Carb= **Sodium Controlled=** **Vegetarian=**

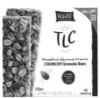

KASHI
TLC Crunchy Granola
Bars, Roasted Almond
Crunch
2 bars
180 Calories

KASHI
GoLean Crunchy Protein
& Fiber Bar, Chocolate
Peanut
1 bar
190 Calories

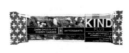

KIND
Plus Bars, Dark Choco-
late Cherry Cashew +
Antioxidants
1 bar
180 Calories

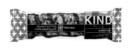

KIND
Plus Bars, Peanut Butter
Dark Chocolate + Protein
1 bar
200 Calories

KRAFT
Macaroni and Cheese
Original Cup
1 container
220 Calories

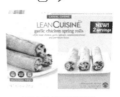

LEAN CUISINE
Casual Cuisine Garlic
Chicken Spring Rolls
1 package
200 Calories

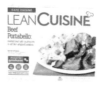

LEAN CUISINE
Cafe Cuisine Beef
Portabello
1 meal
210 Calories

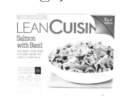

LEAN CUISINE
Spa Cuisine Salmon with
Basil
1 meal
210 Calories

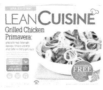

LEAN CUISINE
Spa Cuisine Grilled
Chicken Primavera
1 meal
220 Calories

LEAN CUISINE
Cafe Cuisine Shrimp and
Angel Hair Pasta
1 meal
230 Calories

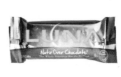

LUNA
Nutz Over Chocolate
1 bar
180 Calories

NATURE'S PATH
Organic Frosted Toaster
Pastries, Strawberry
1 pastry
210 Calories

Build-a-Meal 200-Calorie
Lunch Sides and Afternoon Snacks

Low Carb= Sodium Controlled= Vegetarian=

OREIDA
Bagel Bites Cheese
and Pepperoni
4 pieces
190 Calories

PERDUE
Short Cuts Carved
Chicken Breast, Original
Roasted
1 6-ounce package
225 Calories

PROGRESSO
Traditional Chicken
and Herb Dumplings
1 can
200 Calories

READY PAC
Italiano Bistro Salad
1 package
200 Calories

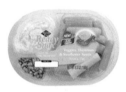

READY PAC
Ready Snax Veggies,
Hummus & Sunflower
Seeds Snack Pac
1 package
220 Calories

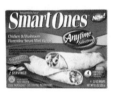

READY PAC
Chicken Caesar
Bistro Salad
1 package
230 Calories

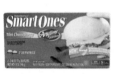

SMART ONES
Mini Cheeseburgers
1 burger
200 Calories

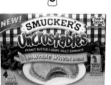

SMART ONES
Chicken and Mushroom
Florentine Smart
Mini Wraps
2 wraps
220 Calories

SMART ONES
Chicken Oriental
1 meal
230 Calories

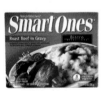

SMART ONES
Roast Beef in Gravy
1 meal
230 Calories

SMART ONES
Angel Hair Marinara
1 meal
230 Calories

SMUCKER'S
Uncrustables Peanut
Butter and Grape Jelly on
Whole Wheat Bread
1 sandwich
210 Calories

Build-a-Meal 200-Calorie
Lunch Sides and Afternoon Snacks

Low Carb=  **Sodium Controlled=** **Vegetarian=**

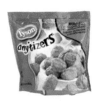

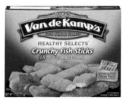

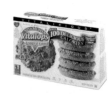

STONYFIELD
Super Smoothie Straw-
berry Banana
1 10-ounce bottle
230 Calories

TYSON
AnyTizers Buffalo Style
Boneless Chicken Bites
8 pieces
190 Calories

VAN DE KAMP'S
Healthy Selects Crunchy
Fish Sticks
6 sticks
180 Calories

VITALICIOUS
Apple Crumb VitaTops
2 muffins
200 Calories

WEIGHT WATCHERS
Three Cheese Macaroni
1 meal
220 Calories

Build-a-Meal 250-Calorie
Lunch Sides and Afternoon Snacks

Low Carb= 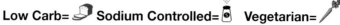 **Sodium Controlled=** **Vegetarian=**

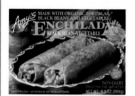

AMY'S
Black Bean and Vegetable
Enchilada
1 container
240 Calories

AMY'S
Medium Southwestern
Black Bean Chili
½ can
240 Calories

AMY'S
Gluten Free Non Dairy
Burrito
1 burrito
240 Calories

AMY'S
Light in Sodium Traditional
Refried Beans
½ can
245 Calories

AMY'S
Traditional Refried Beans
½ can
245 Calories

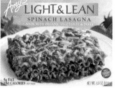

AMY'S
Light & Lean Spinach
Lasagna
1 container
250 Calories

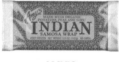

AMY'S
Indian Samosa Wrap
1 wrap
250 Calories

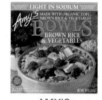

AMY'S
Light in Sodium Brown
Rice & Vegetables Bowl
1 bowl
260 Calories

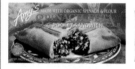

AMY'S
Spinach Feta in a Pocket
Sandwich
1 sandwich
260 Calories

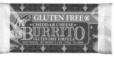

AMY'S
Gluten Free Cheddar
Burrito
1 burrito
260 Calories

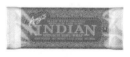

AMY'S
Indian Spinach Tofu Wrap
1 wrap
270 Calories

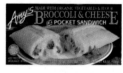

AMY'S
Broccoli & Cheese in a
Pocket Sandwich
1 sandwich
270 Calories

Build-a-Meal 250-Calorie Lunch Sides and Afternoon Snacks

Low Carb= **Sodium Controlled=** **Vegetarian=**

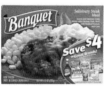

BANQUET
Salisbury Steak Meal
1 meal
250 Calories

BLUE DIAMOND
Wasabi and Soy Sauce
Almonds
1 1.5-ounce bag
255 Calories

BLUE DIAMOND
Jalapeño Smokehouse
Almonds
1 1.5-ounce bag
255 Calories

BLUE DIAMOND
Salt 'n Vinegar Almonds
1 1.5-ounce bag
255 Calories

CAMPBELL'S
Healthy Request Sirloin
Burger with Country Veg-
etables Chunky Soup
1 can
240 Calories

CAMPBELL'S
Healthy Request Classic
Chicken Noodle
Chunky Soup
Microwaveable Bowl
1 bowl
240 Calories

CAMPBELL'S
Slow Roasted Beef with
Mushrooms Chunky Soup
1 can
240 Calories

CAMPBELL'S
Healthy Request Select
Harvest Mexican-Style
Chicken Tortilla Soup
1 can
240 Calories

CAMPBELL'S
Cream of Mushroom
Condensed Soup
1 can
250 Calories

CAMPBELL'S
Cheddar Cheese
Condensed Soup
1 can
250 Calories

CAMPBELL'S
Healthy Request Veg-
etable Condensed Soup
1 can
250 Calories

CAMPBELL'S
Broccoli Cheese
Condensed Soup
1 can
250 Calories

ALL-AMERICAN DIET

Build-a-Meal 250-Calorie Lunch Sides and Afternoon Snacks

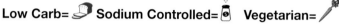 Low Carb= Sodium Controlled= Vegetarian=

CAMPBELL'S
Cream of Shrimp
Condensed Soup
1 can
250 Calories

CAMPBELL'S
Beef with Country Veg-
etables Chunky Soup
1 can
260 Calories

CAMPBELL'S
Select Harvest Italian-
Style Wedding Soup
1 can
260 Calories

CAMPBELL'S
Cream of Onion
Condensed Soup
1 can
268 Calories

DEL MONTE
Red Grapefruit Ready to
Enjoy
1 bowl
270 Calories

DOLE
Light Caesar Kit
1 package
270 Calories

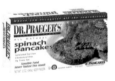

DR. PRAEGER'S
Spinach Pancakes
3 pancakes
240 Calories

EL MONTEREY
Chicken & Cheese
Taquitos
2 taquitos
240 Calories

GORTON'S
Garlic Butter Shrimp Bowl
1 bowl
260 Calories

HEALTHY CHOICE
All Natural Creamy Basil
Pesto
1 meal
240 Calories

HEALTHY CHOICE
All Natural Tortellini
Primavera Parmesan
1 meal
240 Calories

HEALTHY CHOICE
Café Steamers Thai Style
Chicken & Vegetables
1 meal
240 Calories

Build-a-Meal 250-Calorie
Lunch Sides and Afternoon Snacks

Low Carb= **Sodium Controlled=** **Vegetarian=**

HEALTHY CHOICE
Café Steamers Balsamic
Garlic Chicken
1 meal
250 Calories

HEALTHY CHOICE
Steaming Entrees Garlic
Herb Shrimp
1 meal
260 Calories

HEALTHY CHOICE
Canned Soup Garden
Vegetable
1 can
260 Calories

HEALTHY CHOICE
Microwaveable Bowls
Tomato Basil
1 bowl
260 Calories

HEALTHY CHOICE
Café Steamers Chicken
Red Pepper Alfredo
1 meal
260 Calories

HEALTHY CHOICE
Café Steamers Cajun
Style Chicken and Shrimp
1 meal
260 Calories

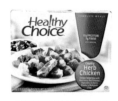

HEALTHY CHOICE
Complete Meals Country
Herb Chicken
1 meal
270 Calories

HEALTHY CHOICE
Café Steamers Grilled
Basil Chicken
1 meal
270 Calories

HEALTHY CHOICE
All Natural Lobster
Cheese Ravioli
1 meal
270 Calories

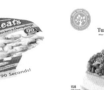

HORMEL
Compleats Chicken and
Dumplings
1 package
260 Calories

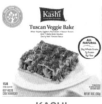

KASHI
Tuscan Veggie Bake
1 meal
260 Calories

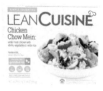

LEAN CUISINE
Simple Favorites Chicken
Chow Mein
1 meal
240 Calories

ALL-AMERICAN DIET

Build-a-Meal 250-Calorie
Lunch Sides and Afternoon Snacks

Low Carb= Sodium Controlled= Vegetarian=

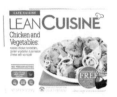

LEAN CUISINE
Cafe Cuisine Chicken and
Vegetables
1 meal
240 Calories

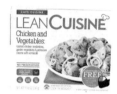

LEAN CUISINE
Cafe Cuisine Chicken and
Vegetables
1 container
240 Calories

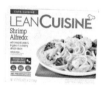

LEAN CUISINE
Cafe Cuisine Shrimp
Alfredo
1 meal
250 Calories

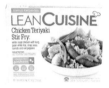

LEAN CUISINE
Simple Favorites Chicken
Teriyaki Stir Fry
1 meal
250 Calories

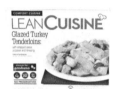

LEAN CUISINE
Comfort Cuisine Glazed
Turkey Tenderloins
1 meal
250 Calories

LEAN CUISINE
Market Creations Shrimp
Scampi
1 container
250 Calories

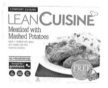

LEAN CUISINE
Comfort Cuisine Meatloaf
with Mashed Potatoes
1 meal
250 Calories

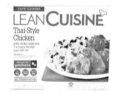

LEAN CUISINE
Cafe Cuisine Thai-Syle
Chicken
1 meal
260 Calories

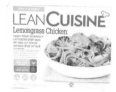

LEAN CUISINE
Spa Cuisine Lemongrass
Chicken
1 meal
260 Calories

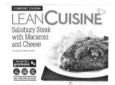

LEAN CUISINE
Comfort Cuisine Salisbury
Steak with Macaroni
and Cheese
1 meal
260 Calories

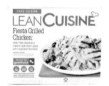

LEAN CUISINE
Cafe Cuisine Fiesta Grilled
Chicken
1 meal
260 Calories

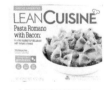

LEAN CUISINE
Simple Favorites Pasta
Romano with Bacon
1 meal
260 Calories

LUNCH SIDES AND AFTERNOON SNACKS

Build-a-Meal 250-Calorie
Lunch Sides and Afternoon Snacks

Low Carb= **Sodium Controlled=** **Vegetarian=**

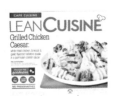

LEAN CUISINE
Cafe Cuisine Grilled
Chicken Caesar
1 container
260 Calories

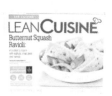

LEAN CUISINE
Spa Cuisine Butternut
Squash Ravioli
1 container
260 Calories

LEAN CUISINE
Market Creations Asiago
Cheese Tortelloni
1 meal
270 Calories

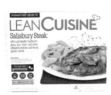

LEAN CUISINE
Dinnertime Selects
Salisbury Steak
1 container
270 Calories

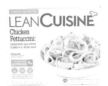

LEAN CUISINE
Simple Favorites Chicken
Fettuccini
1 container
270 Calories

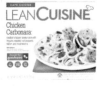

LEAN CUISINE
Cafe Cuisine Chicken
Carbonara
1 meal
270 Calories

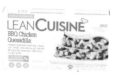

LEAN CUISINE
Simple Favorites BBQ
Chicken Quesadilla
1 meal
270 Calories

LEAN POCKETS
Culinary Creations Grilled
Chicken Mushroom &
Spinach
1 piece
240 Calories

LEAN POCKETS
Mexican Style Chicken
Fiesta
1 piece
240 Calories

LEAN POCKETS
Culinary Creations Garlic
Chicken White Pizza
1 piece
260 Calories

LEAN POCKETS
Whole Grain Turkey
Broccoli & Cheese
1 piece
260 Calories

LEAN POCKETS
Pizzeria Four Cheese in
Seasoned Herb Crust
1 piece
270 Calories

Build-a-Meal 250-Calorie
Lunch Sides and Afternoon Snacks

Low Carb= Sodium Controlled= Vegetarian=

LEAN POCKETS
Culinary Creations
Chicken Bacon Dijon
1 piece
270 Calories

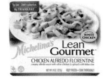

MICHELINA'S
Lean Gourmet Chicken
Alfredo Florentine
1 package
260 Calories

MORNINGSTAR FARMS
Three Bean Chili
1 package
270 Calories

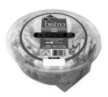

READY PAC
Chef Bistro Salad
1 package
270 Calories

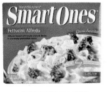

SMART ONES
Fettucini Alfredo
1 meal
240 Calories

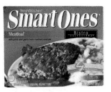

SMART ONES
Meatloaf
1 meal
240 Calories

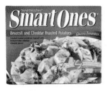

SMART ONES
Broccoli and Cheddar
Roasted Potatoes
1 meal
240 Calories

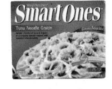

SMART ONES
Tuna Noodle Gratin
1 meal
250 Calories

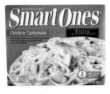

SMART ONES
Chicken Carbonara
1 meal
260 Calories

SMART ONES
Cheese Pizza Minis
4 pizzas
270 Calories

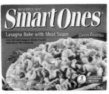

SMART ONES
Lasagna Bake with Meat
Sauce
1 meal
270 Calories

SPAM
Single Classic
1 package
250 Calories

LUNCH SIDES AND AFTERNOON SNACKS

133

Build-a-Meal 250-Calorie
Lunch Sides and Afternoon Snacks

Low Carb= 🍞 **Sodium Controlled=** 🧂 **Vegetarian=** 🌿

STOUFFER'S
Homestyle Classics
Baked Chicken Breast
1 meal
250 calories

DIET DETECTIVE WHAT YOU NEED TO KNOW

KNOCK OUT

Knock out your excuses with excuse busting. Come up with Excuse Busters and Plan Bs. Punch holes in your excuses until they are no longer airtight. Create a list of all your excuses for not eating healthy and exercising more. Then come up with counterarguments for every single excuse you may have for NOT achieving your goals.

Build-a-Meal
350-Calorie Dinner Entrées

Low Carb= **Sodium Controlled=** **Vegetarian=**

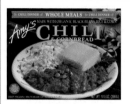

AMY'S
Whole Meals Chili &
Cornbread
1 meal
340 Calories

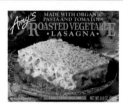

AMY'S
Roasted Vegetable
Lasagna
1 container
350 Calories

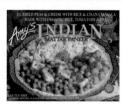

AMY'S
Indian Mattar Paneer
1 meal
370 Calories

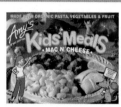

AMY'S
Mac N' Cheese Kids Meal
1 meal
370 Calories

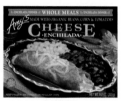

AMY'S
Whole Meals Cheese
Enchilada
1 meal
370 Calories

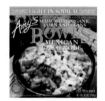

AMY'S
Light in Sodium Mexican
Casserole Bowl
1 bowl
370 Calories

AMY'S
Light in Sodium
Lentil Soup
1 can
370 Calories

ANNIE CHUN'S
Vegetarian Spicy Veg-
etable Mini Wontons
1 package
360 Calories

BANQUET
Chicken Pot Pie
1 pie
370 Calories

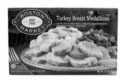

BOSTON MARKET
Turkey Breast Medallions
Meal
1 meal
360 Calories

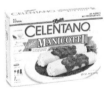

CELENTANO
Manicotti
1 meal
370 Calories

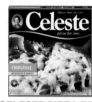

**CELESTE PIZZA FOR
ONE**
Original
1 pizza
340 Calories

Build-a-Meal
350-Calorie Dinner Entrées

Low Carb= 🍞 **Sodium Controlled=** 🧂 **Vegetarian=** 🌿

CELESTE PIZZA FOR ONE
Vegetable
1 pizza
350 Calories
🌿

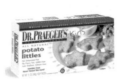

DR. PRAEGER'S
Potato Littles
6 pieces
360 Calories
🧂 🌿

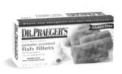

DR. PRAEGER'S
Potato Crusted Fish Fillets
4 fillets
360 Calories
🌿

GREEN GIANT
Garden Vegetable Medley
1 package
350 Calories

GREEN GIANT
Roasted Potatoes with Garlic & Herb Sauce
1 package
360 Calories
🌿

HEALTHY CHOICE
Café Steamers Sweet Sesame Chicken
1 meal
340 Calories
🧂

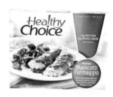

HEALTHY CHOICE
Complete Meals Marinara Manicotti Formaggio
1 container
350 Calories
🧂 🌿

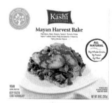

KASHI
Mayan Harvest Bake
1 container
340 Calories
🧂 🌿

LEAN CUISINE
Casual Cuisine Deluxe Pizza
1 pizza
340 Calories
🧂

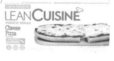

LEAN CUISINE
Simple Favorites Cheese French Bread Pizza
1 meal
340 Calories
🧂

LEAN CUISINE
Casual Cuisine Four Cheese Pizza
1 pizza
350 Calories
🧂 🌿

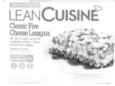

LEAN CUISINE
Simple Favorites Classic Five Cheese Lasagna
1 container
360 Calories
🌿

ALL-AMERICAN DIET

Build-a-Meal
350-Calorie Dinner Entrées

Low Carb= **Sodium Controlled=** 🧂 **Vegetarian=** 🌱

LEAN CUISINE
Casual Cuisine Chicken
Ranch Club Flatbread
Melt
1 meal
370 Calories

PERDUE
Crispy Chicken Strips
4 strips
340 Calories
🧂

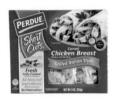

PERDUE
Short Cuts Carved
Chicken Breast Grilled
Italian Style
1 9-ounce package
350 Calories

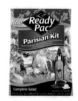

READY PAC
Parisian Kit Complete
Salad
1 bag
350 Calories
🧂

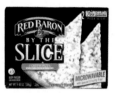

RED BARON
4-Cheese Pizza By the
Slice
1 slice
340 Calories
🌱

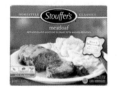

STOUFFER'S
Homestyle Classics
Meatloaf
1 meal
340 Calories

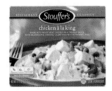

STOUFFER'S
Restaurant Classics
Chicken á la King
1 meal
360 Calories

STOUFFER'S
Corner Bistro Toasted
Sub Philly Style Steak &
Cheese
1 sandwich
370 Calories

STOUFFER'S
Corner Bistro Chicken
Quesadilla Flatbread Melt
1 sandwich
370 Calories

TYSON
Grilled & Ready Fajita
Chicken Breast Strips
1 10-ounce bag
350 Calories

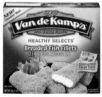

VAN DE KAMP'S
Healthy Selects Breaded
Fish Fillets
4 fillets
360 Calories

Build-a-Meal
400-Calorie Dinner Entrées

Low Carb= 🍞 **Sodium Controlled=** 🧂 **Vegetarian=** 🥕

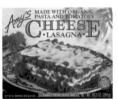

AMY'S
Cheese Lasagna
1 container
380 Calories
🥕

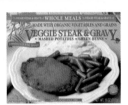

AMY'S
Whole Meals Veggie
Steak & Gravy
1 meal
380 Calories
🥕

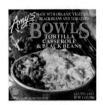

AMY'S
Tortilla Casserole & Black
Beans Bowl
1 bowl
390 Calories
🥕

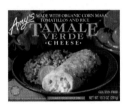

AMY'S
Cheese Tamale Verde
1 meal
400 Calories
🥕

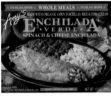

AMY'S
Whole Meals Enchilada
Verde
1 meal
400 Calories
🥕

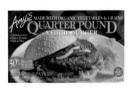

AMY'S
Quarter Pound Veggie
Burger
2 burgers
400 Calories
🥕

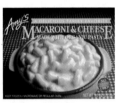

AMY'S
Macaroni & Cheese
1 container
410 Calories
🧂 🥕

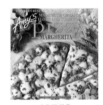

AMY'S
Margherita Pizza
½ pizza
420 Calories
🥕

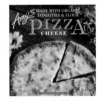

AMY'S
Single Serve Cheese
Pizza
1 pizza
420 Calories
🥕

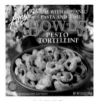

AMY'S
Pesto Tortellini Bowl
1 bowl
430 Calories
🥕

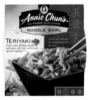

ANNIE CHUN'S
Teriyaki Noodle Bowl
1 bowl
400 Calories
🥕

BANQUET
Turkey Pot Pie
1 pie
380 Calories

Build-a-Meal
400-Calorie Dinner Entrées

Low Carb= 🍞 **Sodium Controlled=** 🧂 **Vegetarian=** 🥕

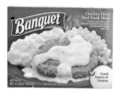

BANQUET
Chicken Fried Beef Steak
Meal
1 meal
390 Calories

BANQUET
Beef Pot Pie
1 pie
390 Calories

BARBER FOODS
Fit and Flavorful Broc-
coli and Cheese Stuffed
Chicken Breast
2 pieces
380 Calories

CAMPBELL'S
Creamy Chicken &
Dumplings Chunky Soup
Microwaveable Bowl
1 bowl
380 Calories

CAMPBELL'S
Chicken Broccoli Cheese
with Potato Chunky Soup
1 can
420 Calories

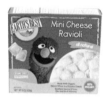

EARTH'S BEST
Mini Cheese Ravioli
1 meal
380 Calories
🧂 🥕

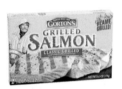

GORTON'S
Classic Grilled Salmon
Fillets
4 fillets
400 Calories
🍞

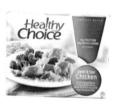

HEALTHY CHOICE
Complete Meals Sweet &
Sour Chicken
1 meal
420 Calories
🧂

HORMEL
Vegetarian Chili with
Beans
1 can
380 Calories
🥕

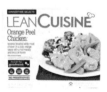

LEAN CUISINE
Dinnertime Selects Or-
ange Peel Chicken
1 meal
380 Calories

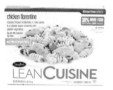

LEAN CUISINE
Dinnertime Selects
Chicken Florentine
1 container
410 Calories

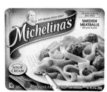

MICHELINA'S
Traditional Recipes Swed-
ish Meatballs with Gravy
& Pasta
1 package
380 Calories

Build-a-Meal
400-Calorie Dinner Entrées

Low Carb= Sodium Controlled= Vegetarian=

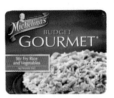

MICHELINA'S
Budget Gourmet Stir Fry
Rice & Vegetables
1 package
390 Calories

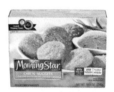

MORNINGSTAR FARMS
Chik'n Nuggets
8 nuggets
380 Calories

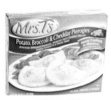

MRS. T'S
Potato Broccoli & Ched-
dar Pierogies
6 pieces
380 Calories

NISSIN
Top Ramen, Chicken
Flavor
1 package
380 Calories

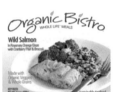

ORGANIC BISTRO
Savory Turkey
1 meal
370 Calories

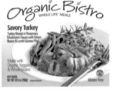

ORGANIC BISTRO
Wild Salmon
1 meal
390 Calories

READY PAC
Santa Fe Caesar Com-
plete Salad
1 bag
375 Calories

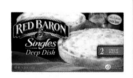

RED BARON
Singles Deep Dish
Cheese Pizzas
1 pizza
400 Calories

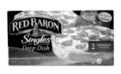

RED BARON
Singles Deep Dish Pep-
peroni Pizzas
1 pizza
420 Calories

SEEDS OF CHANGE
Tapovan White Basmati
Rice
1 package
420 Calories

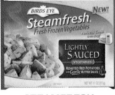

STEAMFRESH
Lightly Sauced Vegetables
Roasted Red Potatoes
with Garlic Butter Sauce
1 package
380 Calories

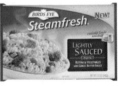

STEAMFRESH
Lightly Sauced Pasta
Rotini & Vegetables with
Garlic Butter Sauce
1 package
420 Calories

ALL-AMERICAN DIET

Build-a-Meal
400-Calorie Dinner Entrées

Low Carb=  **Sodium Controlled=** 🧂 **Vegetarian=** 🌿

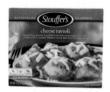

STOUFFER'S
Restaurant Classics
Cheese Ravioli
1 meal
380 Calories
🌿

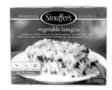

STOUFFER'S
Homestyle Classics Vegetable Lasagna
1 meal
390 Calories
🌿

STOUFFER'S
Corner Bistro Toasted
Sub Meatball Italiano
1 sandwich
400 Calories

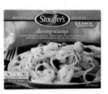

STOUFFER'S
Restaurant Selects
Shrimp Scampi, Large
Size
1 meal
400 Calories

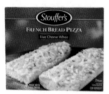

STOUFFER'S
5 Cheese White French
Bread Pizza
1 piece
420 Calories
🌿

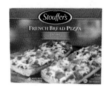

STOUFFER'S
Deluxe French Bread
Pizza
1 piece
430 Calories

TYSON
Crispy Chicken Strips
6 pieces
380 Calories

TYSON
Grilled & Ready Oven
Roasted Diced Chicken
Breast
1 10-ounce bag
385 Calories

UNCLE BEN'S
Ready Whole Grain Medley Roasted Garlic
1 package
400 Calories
🧂 🌿

UNCLE BEN'S
Cajun Style Ready Rice
1 package
420 Calories
🌿

DINNER ENTRÉES

Build-a-Meal
450-Calorie Dinner Entrées

Low Carb= 🍞 **Sodium Controlled=** 🧂 **Vegetarian=** 🥕

AMY'S
Broccoli & Spinach White
Pizza
½ pizza
435 Calories
🥕

AMY'S
Cheese Pizza
½ pizza
435 Calories
🥕

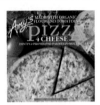

AMY'S
Four Cheese Pizza
½ pizza
435 Calories
🥕

AMY'S
Soy Cheeze Pizza
½ pizza
435 Calories
🥕

AMY'S
Light in Sodium Single
Serve Spinach Pizza
1 pizza
440 Calories
🧂 🥕

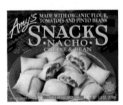

AMY'S
Nacho Cheese & Bean
Snacks
1 box
440 Calories
🥕

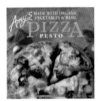

AMY'S
Single Serve Pesto Pizza
1 pizza
440 Calories
🥕

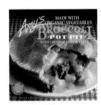

AMY'S
Broccoli Pot Pie
1 pie
460 Calories
🥕

AMY'S
Non-Dairy Cheeze Rice
Crust Single Serve Pizza
1 pizza
460 Calories
🥕

AMY'S
Pesto Pizza
½ pizza
465 Calories
🥕

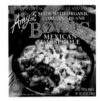

AMY'S
Mexican Casserole Bowl
1 bowl
470 Calories
🥕

ANNIE CHUN'S
Pad Thai Noodle Bowl
1 bowl
460 Calories
🥕

ALL-AMERICAN DIET

Build-a-Meal
450-Calorie Dinner Entrées

Low Carb= 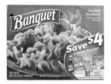 **Sodium Controlled=** 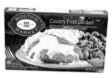 **Vegetarian=** [pepper icon]

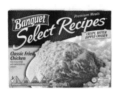

BANQUET
Swedish Meatballs
1 meal
440 Calories

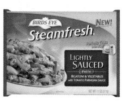

BANQUET
Select Recipes Crispy
Batter Dipped Chicken
1 meal
440 Calories

[BIRDS EYE image]

BIRDS EYE
Steamfresh Lightly
Sauced Pasta Rigatoni &
Vegetables with Tomato
Parmesan Sauce
1 package
440 Calories

[BOSTON MARKET image]

BOSTON MARKET
Country Fried
Chicken Meal
1 meal
470 Calories

CAMPBELL'S
Healthy Kids SpaghettiOs
with Sliced Franks
1 can
440 Calories

CAMPBELL'S
Green Pea
Condensed Soup
1 can
450 Calories
[pepper icon]

CAMPBELL'S
Split Pea with Ham
Condensed Soup
1 can
450 Calories

CAMPBELL'S
New England Clam
Chowder Chunky Soup
1 can
460 Calories

CHEF BOYARDEE
Beef Ravioli Microwave-
able Big Size Bowl
1 bowl
440 Calories

DOLE
Asian Island Crunch Kit
1 bag
456 Calories
[pepper icon]

DOLE
Southwest Salad Kit
1 bag
460 Calories
[pepper icon]

HORMEL
Microwaveable Bowls
Chili with Beans
1 bowl
440 Calories

Build-a-Meal
450-Calorie Dinner Entrées

Low Carb= **Sodium Controlled=** **Vegetarian=**

JIMMY DEAN
Biscuit Sandwiches Sausage Egg & Cheese
1 sandwich
440 Calories

OSCAR MAYER
Deli Creations Hot Sandwich Melts Honey Ham & Swiss
1 package
440 Calories

SEEDS OF CHANGE
Rishikesh Whole Grain Brown Basmati Rice
1 package
440 Calories

SEEDS OF CHANGE
Dharamsala Aromatic Indian Rice Blend
1 package
460 Calories

SIMPLY ASIA
Spicy Mongolian Noodle Bowl
1 bowl
450 Calories

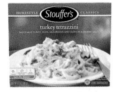

STOUFFER'S
Homestyle Classics Turkey Tetrazzini
1 meal
450 Calories

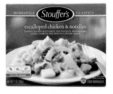

STOUFFER'S
Homestyle Classics Escalloped Chicken & Noodles
1 meal
450 Calories

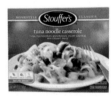

STOUFFER'S
Homestyle Classics Tuna Noodle Casserole
1 meal
450 Calories

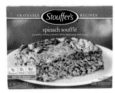

STOUFFER'S
Craveable Recipes Spinach Soufflé
1 meal
450 Calories

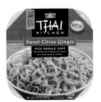

THAI KITCHEN
Sweet Citrus Ginger Rice Noodle Cart
1 package
440 Calories

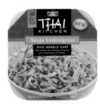

THAI KITCHEN
Tangy Lemongrass Rice Noodle Cart
1 package
450 Calories

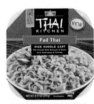

THAI KITCHEN
Pad Thai Rice Noodle Cart
1 package
460 Calories

ALL-AMERICAN DIET

Build-a-Meal
450-Calorie Dinner Entrées

Low Carb= 🍞 **Sodium Controlled=** 🧂 **Vegetarian=** 🌿

UNCLE BEN'S
Ready Rice Chicken Flavored Whole Grain Brown
1 package
440 Calories

UNCLE BEN'S
Ready Whole Grain Medley Brown & Wild
1 package
440 Calories
🌿

UNCLE BEN'S
Ready Whole Grain Medley Santa Fe
1 package
440 Calories
🌿

UNCLE BEN'S
Ready Whole Grain Medley Vegetable Harvest
1 package
440 Calories
🌿

UNCLE BEN'S
Ready Rice Basmati
1 package
440 Calories
🧂 🌿

UNCLE BEN'S
Ready Rice Long Grain & Wild
1 package
440 Calories
🌿

UNCLE BEN'S
Ready Rice Roasted Chicken
1 package
440 Calories

UNCLE BEN'S
Ready Rice Rice Pilaf
1 package
440 Calories
🌿

Build-a-Meal
500-Calorie Dinner Entrées

Low Carb= 🍞 **Sodium Controlled=** 🧂 **Vegetarian=** 🥄

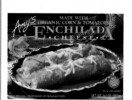

AMY'S
Cheese Enchilada
1 meal
480 Calories
🥄

AMY'S
Light in Sodium Refried
Black Beans
1 can
490 Calories
🧂 🥄

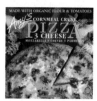

AMY'S
3 Cheese Cornmeal
Crust Pizza
½ pizza
510 Calories
🥄

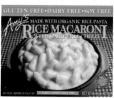

AMY'S
Rice Macaroni with Dairy
Free Cheeze
1 meal
520 Calories
🥄

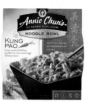

ANNIE CHUN'S
Kung Pao Noodle Bowl
1 bowl
480 Calories
🥄

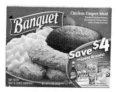

BANQUET
Chicken Fingers Meal
1 meal
480 Calories

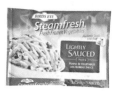

BIRDS EYE
Steamfresh Lightly
Sauced Penne and
Vegetables with
Alfredo Sauce
1 bag
520 Calories

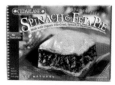

CEDARLANE
Spinach & Feta Pie
1 package
520 Calories
🥄

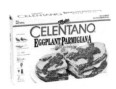

CELENTANO
Eggplant Parmigiana
1 meal
520 Calories
🥄

DOLE
Perfect Harvest Kit
1 bag
490 Calories
🧂 🥄

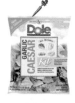

DOLE
Garlic Caesar Kit
1 bag
525 Calories
🥄

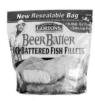

GORTON'S
Beer Battered Fish Fillets
4 fillets
500 Calories

ALL-AMERICAN DIET

Build-a-Meal
500-Calorie Dinner Entrées

Low Carb= Sodium Controlled= Vegetarian=

HORMEL
Hot Chili with Beans
1 can
520 Calories

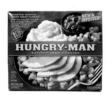

HUNGRY MAN
Roasted Carved White
Meat Turkey
1 meal
540 Calories

SEEDS OF CHANGE
Uyuni Quinoa & Whole
Grain Brown Rice
1 package
480 Calories

SEEDS OF CHANGE
Arroz Hispaniola
Caribbean Red Beans &
Brown Rice
1 package
500 Calories

SEEDS OF CHANGE
Tigris A Mixture of Seven
Whole Grains
1 package
520 Calories

SIMPLY ASIA
Spicy Kung Pao Noodle
Bowl
1 bowl
480 Calories

SIMPLY ASIA
Sweet & Sour Chow Mein
Take Out
1 box
500 Calories

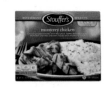

STOUFFER'S
Restaurant Selects Mon-
terey Chicken
1 meal
530 Calories

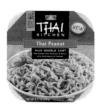

THAI KITCHEN
Thai Peanut Rice Noodle
Cart
1 package
520 Calories

TYSON
Grilled & Ready Seasoned
Steak Strips
1 10-ounce bag
490 Calories

UNCLE BEN'S
Ready Rice Whole Grain
Brown
1 package
480 Calories

UNCLE BEN'S
Ready Rice Jasmine
1 package
500 Calories

Build-a-Meal
600-Calorie Dinner Entrées

Low Carb= **Sodium Controlled=** **Vegetarian=**

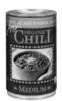

AMY'S
Light in Sodium Medium Chili
1 can
560 Calories

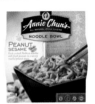

ANNIE CHUN'S
Peanut Sesame Noodle Bowl
1 bowl
560 Calories

ANNIE CHUN'S
Pork and Ginger Mini Wontons
1 container
600 Calories

ANNIE CHUN'S
Garlic Scallion Noodle Bowl
1 bowl
620 Calories

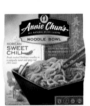

ANNIE CHUN'S
Korean Sweet Chili Noodle Bowl
1 bowl
640 Calories

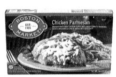

BOSTON MARKET
Chicken Parmesan Meal
1 meal
620 Calories

DOLE
Hearty Italian Kit
1 package
552 Calories

DOLE
Ultimate Caesar Kit
1 package
552 Calories

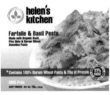

HELEN'S KITCHEN
Farfalle & Basil Pesto
1 meal
590 Calories

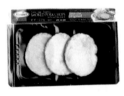

HORMEL
Smoked Pork Chops Thick Cut Original
2 chops
560 Calories

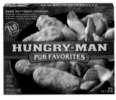

HUNGRY MAN
Beer Battered Chicken
1 meal
560 Calories

HUNGRY MAN
Salisbury Steak
1 meal
600 Calories

ALL-AMERICAN DIET

148

Build-a-Meal
600-Calorie Dinner Entrées

Low Carb= **Sodium Controlled=** 🧂 **Vegetarian=** 🌿

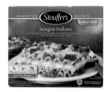

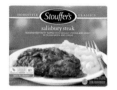

STOUFFER'S
Homestyle Selects
Lasagna Italiano, Large
Size
1 meal
580 Calories

STOUFFER'S
Homestyle Classics
Salisbury Steak
1 meal
630 Calories

Build-a-Meal
50-Calorie Dinner Sides

Low Carb= 🥖 **Sodium Controlled=** 🧂 **Vegetarian=** 🌿

AMY'S
Low Fat Vegetable Barley
Soup
½ can
70 Calories
🌿

CAMPBELL'S
Vegetable Beef Soup at
Hand
1 container
70 Calories

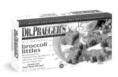

DR. PRAEGER'S
Broccoli Littles
2 pieces
40 Calories
🧂 🌿

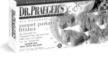

DR. PRAEGER'S
Sweet Potato Littles
2 pieces
60 Calories
🧂 🌿

GREAT VALUE
Fat Free Smoked Turkey
Breast
2 slices
50 Calories
🥖 🧂

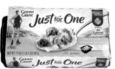

GREEN GIANT
Just for One Broccoli &
Cheese
1 container
40 Calories
🧂 🌿

HILLSHIRE FARM
Brown Sugar Baked Ham
6 slices
60 Calories
🥖

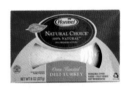

HORMEL
Natural Choice Oven
Roasted Deli Turkey
3 slices
60 Calories
🥖 🧂

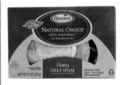

HORMEL
Natural Choice Honey Deli
Ham
4 slices
70 Calories
🥖

SARGENTO
Reduced Fat Sharp
Cheddar Cheese Sticks
1 stick
60 Calories
🥖 🧂 🌿

**STRETCH ISLAND
FRUIT CO.**
All-Natural Fruit Strip,
Summer Strawberry
1 strip
45 Calories
🧂

WEIGHT WATCHERS
Reduced Fat Singles,
American
1 slice
45 Calories
🥖 🧂 🌿

ALL-AMERICAN DIET

Build-a-Meal
100-Calorie Dinner Sides

Low Carb= Sodium Controlled= Vegetarian=

ALEXIA
Classic French Rolls
1 roll
100 Calories

ALEXIA
Focaccia Rolls
1 roll
120 Calories

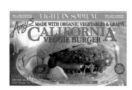

AMY'S
Light in Sodium California
Veggie Burger
1 burger
100 Calories

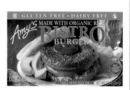

AMY'S
Bistro Burger
1 burger
110 Calories

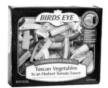

BIRDS EYE
Tuscan Vegetables in an
Herbed Tomato Sauce
1 package
125 Calories

BOCA
All American Classic
Meatless Burgers
1 burger
120 Calories

BUMBLE BEE
Prime Fillet Chicken
Breast, Garlic and Herb
1 package
110 Calories

CAMPBELL'S
Select Harvest Light Veg-
etable and Pasta Soup
1 can
120 Calories

CAMPBELL'S
Beefy Mushroom
Condensed Soup
1 can
125 Calories

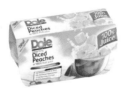

DOLE
Diced Peaches
1 container
80 Calories

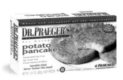

DR. PRAEGER'S
Potato Pancakes
1 pancake
100 Calories

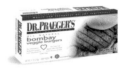

DR. PRAEGER'S
Bombay Veggie Burgers
1 burger
110 Calories

Build-a-Meal
100-Calorie Dinner Sides

Low Carb= Sodium Controlled= Vegetarian=

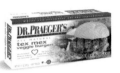

DR. PRAEGER'S
Tex Mex Veggie Burgers
1 burger
110 Calories

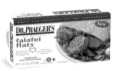

DR. PRAEGER'S
Falafel Flats
3 pieces
110 Calories

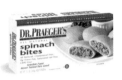

DR. PRAEGER'S
Spinach Bites
2 pieces
110 Calories

GARDENBURGER
Veggie Medley Veggie
Burgers, Vegan
1 patty
100 Calories

GARDENBURGER
Portabella Veggie Burgers
1 patty
100 Calories

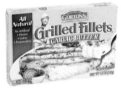

GORTON'S
Grilled Garlic Butter Fish
Fillets
1 fillet
100 Calories

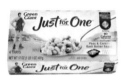

GREEN GIANT
Just for One Peas and
Corn in Basil Butter Sauce
1 container
80 Calories

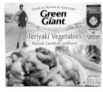

GREEN GIANT
Teriyaki Vegetables
1 package
100 Calories

GREEN GIANT
Steamers Healthy Colors
Farmer's Blend
1 package
100 Calories

GREEN GIANT
Baby Vegetable Medley
1 package
120 Calories

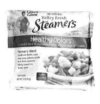

GREEN GIANT
Steamers Healthy Colors
Nature's Blend
1 package
120 Calories

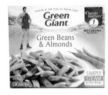

GREEN GIANT
Green Beans and
Almonds
1 package
125 Calories

Build-a-Meal
100-Calorie Dinner Sides

Low Carb=   Sodium Controlled=   Vegetarian=

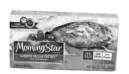

MORNINGSTAR FARMS
Garden Veggie Patties
1 patty
110 Calories

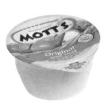

MOTT'S
Original Apple Sauce
1 4-ounce container
100 Calories

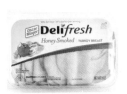

OSCAR MAYER
Deli Fresh Honey Smoked
Turkey Breast
½ 9-ounce package
125 Calories

PIRATE'S BOOTY
Sour Cream & Onion Rice
and Corn Puffs
1-ounce bag
130 Calories

POP CHIPS
Cheddar Potato
1 0.8-ounce bag
100 Calories

POP CHIPS
Sea Salt & Vinegar Potato
1 0.8-ounce bag
100 Calories

PRINGLES
Baked Wheat Stix,
Cheese
1 package
90 Calories

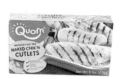

QUORN
Naked Chik'n Cutlets
1 cutlet
80 Calories

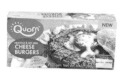

QUORN
Cheese Burgers
1 burger
100 Calories

SARGENTO
Mild Cheddar Cubes
7 cubes
120 Calories

STONYFIELD
0% Fat Pomegranate
Raspberry Acai Smooth
and Creamy
1 container
120 Calories

STONYFIELD
Oikos Greek Yogurt
Honey
1 container
120 Calories

Build-a-Meal
150-Calorie Dinner Sides

Low Carb= **Sodium Controlled=** **Vegetarian=**

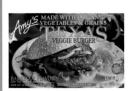

AMY'S
Texas Veggie Burger
1 burger
140 Calories

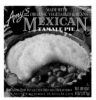

AMY'S
Mexican Tamale Pie
1 pie
150 Calories

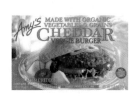

AMY'S
Cheddar Veggie Burger
1 burger
160 Calories

AMY'S
Shepherd's Pie
1 pie
160 Calories

AMY'S
Fat Free Alphabet Soup
1 can
160 Calories

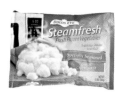

BIRDS EYE
Steamfresh Specially Sea-
soned Garlic Cauliflower
1 bag
160 Calories

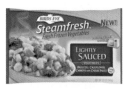

BIRDS EYE
Steamfresh Lightly Sauced
Veg Broccoli, Cauliflower,
Carrots w/Cheese Sauce
1 package
160 Calories

BOCA
Spicy Chicken Meatless
Patties
1 patty
160 Calories

CAMPBELL'S
98% Fat Free Cream of
Mushroom Condensed
Soup
1 can
150 Calories

CAMPBELL'S
Homestyle Chicken
Noodle Condensed Soup
1 can
150 Calories

CAMPBELL'S
Vegetable Beef Micro-
waveable Bowl
1 bowl
160 Calories

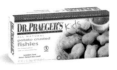

DR. PRAEGER'S
Potato Crusted Fishies
8 pieces
160 Calories

Build-a-Meal
150-Calorie Dinner Sides

Low Carb= 🍞 **Sodium Controlled=** 🧂 **Vegetarian=** 🌿

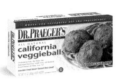

DR. PRAEGER'S
California Veggie Balls
4 pieces
160 Calories
🌿

FRESH EXPRESS
3-Color Deli Coleslaw
1 package
160 Calories
🧂 🌿

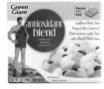

GREEN GIANT
Antioxidant Blend
1 box
140 Calories
🧂 🌿

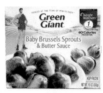

GREEN GIANT
Baby Brussels Sprouts in
Butter Sauce
1 box
150 Calories
🌿

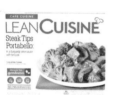

LEAN CUISINE
Cafe Cuisine Steak
Tips Portabello
1 meal
160 Calories
🍞 🧂

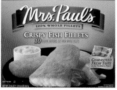

MRS. PAUL'S
Crispy Fish Fillets
1 fillet
145 Calories
🍞

MRS. T'S
Potato & Cheddar
Mini Pierogies
7 pieces
140 Calories
🧂 🌿

PERDUE
Buffalo Style Chicken
Strips
2 strips
140 Calories
🍞

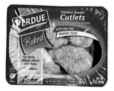

PERDUE
Baked Chicken Breast
Cutlets Italian Style
1 cutlet
160 Calories
🍞

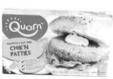

PROGRESSO
Light Beef Pot Roast
1 can
160 Calories

QUORN
Chik'n Patties
1 patty
150 Calories
🧂 🌿

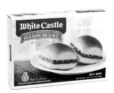

WHITE CASTLE
Microwaveable
Hamburgers
1 burger
140 Calories
🍞 🧂

Build-a-Meal
200-Calorie Dinner Sides

Low Carb= 🍞 Sodium Controlled= 🧂 Vegetarian= 🌿

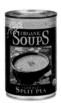

AMY'S
Light in Sodium Low Fat
Split Pea Soup
1 can
200 Calories
🌿

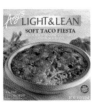

AMY'S
Light & Lean Soft
Taco Fiesta
1 meal
220 Calories
🌿

ANNIE'S
Microwaveable Mac
& Cheese
1 packet
230 Calories
🌿

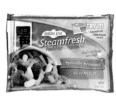

BIRDS EYE
Steamfresh Specially Sea-
soned Asian Medley
1 bag
175 Calories
🌿

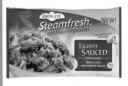

BIRDS EYE
Steamfresh Lightly
Sauced Vegetables
Broccoli with Cheese
Sauce
1 bag
180 Calories

BIRDS EYE
Peas & Pearl Onions
1 box
180 Calories
🌿

BUSH'S
Original Baked Beans
Microwaveable Bowl
1 bowl
224 Calories

CAMPBELL'S
Chicken with Rice
Condensed Soup
1 can
175 Calories

CAMPBELL'S
Healthy Request Cream of
Celery Condensed Soup
1 can
175 Calories
🌿

CAMPBELL'S
Vegetarian Vegetable
Condensed Soup
1 can
180 Calories
🌿

CAMPBELL'S
Healthy Request Cream of
Chicken Condensed Soup
1 can
200 Calories

CAMPBELL'S
Select Harvest Garden
Recipes Minestrone Soup
1 can
200 Calories

ALL-AMERICAN DIET

Build-a-Meal
200-Calorie Dinner Sides

Low Carb= 🍞 **Sodium Controlled=** 🧂 **Vegetarian=** 🌿

CAMPBELL'S
Classic Chicken Noodle
Chunky Soup
Microwaveable Bowl
1 bowl
220 Calories

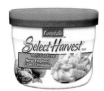

CAMPBELL'S
Select Harvest 98% Fat
Free New England
Clam Chowder
Microwaveable Bowl
1 bowl
220 Calories

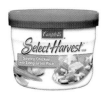

CAMPBELL'S
Select Harvest Savory
Chicken with Long Grain
Rice Microwaveable Bowl
1 bowl
220 Calories

CAMPBELL'S
Beef Rib Roast with
Potatoes & Herbs Chunky
Soup
1 can
220 Calories

CAMPBELL'S
Select Harvest Savory
Chicken with Long Grain
Rice Soup
1 can
220 Calories

CAMPBELL'S
Healthy Request Tomato
Condensed Soup
1 can
225 Calories

🌿

CAMPBELL'S
Vegetable Beef Con-
densed Soup
1 can
225 Calories

**EARTHBOUND FARMS
ORGANIC**
Caesar Grab & Go Salad
1 package
230 Calories

🍞 🧂 🌿

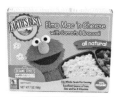

EARTH'S BEST
Elmo Mac 'n Cheese with
Carrots & Broccoli
1 meal
220 Calories

🧂 🌿

FRESH EXPRESS
Caesar Lite Kit
1 package
180 Calories

🍞 🌿

FRESH EXPRESS
House Italian Kit
1 package
210 Calories

🍞 🌿

GREEN GIANT
Healthy Weight
1 box
180 Calories

🧂 🌿

Build-a-Meal
200-Calorie Dinner Sides

Low Carb= **Sodium Controlled=** **Vegetarian=**

HEALTHY CHOICE
Canned Soup
Chicken Noodle
1 can
180 Calories

HEALTHY CHOICE
Steaming Entrées Lemon
Herb Chicken
1 meal
210 Calories

HEALTHY CHOICE
Microwaveable Bowls
Beef Pot Roast
1 bowl
220 Calories

HEALTHY CHOICE
Café Steamers Roasted
Beef Merlot
1 meal
230 Calories

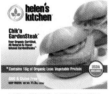

HELEN'S KITCHEN
Chik'n GardenSteak
1 steak
210 Calories

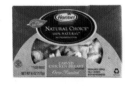

HORMEL
Natural Choice Carved
Chicken Breast Strips
1 package
180 Calories

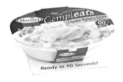

HORMEL
Compleats Chicken
Breast and Gravy
1 package
210 Calories

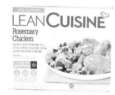

LEAN CUISINE
Spa Cuisine Rosemary
Chicken
1 meal
210 Calories

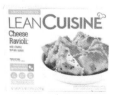

LEAN CUISINE
Simple Favorites
Cheese Ravioli
1 meal
220 Calories

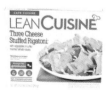

LEAN CUISINE
Cafe Cuisine Three
Cheese Stuffed Rigatoni
1 meal
230 Calories

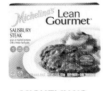

MICHELINA'S
Lean Gourmet Salisbury
Steak
1 package
180 Calories

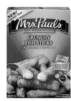

MRS. PAUL'S
Crunchy Fish Sticks
6 sticks
220 Calories

ALL-AMERICAN DIET

Build-a-Meal
200-Calorie Dinner Sides

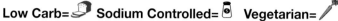

Low Carb= **Sodium Controlled=** **Vegetarian=**

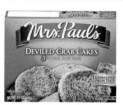

MRS. PAUL'S
Deviled Crab Cakes
1 cake
220 Calories

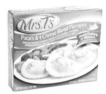

MRS. T'S
Potato & 4 Cheese Blend
Pierogies
3 pieces
220 Calories

PERDUE
Short Cuts Carved
Chicken Breast South-
western Style
1 6-ounce package
225 Calories

TYSON
Grilled & Ready Chicken
Breast Strips
1 6-ounce bag
200 Calories

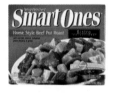

SMART ONES
Homestyle Beef Pot Roast
1 meal
180 Calories

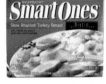

SMART ONES
Slow Roasted Turkey
Breast
1 meal
200 Calories

SMART ONES
Teriyaki Chicken & Veg-
etables
1 meal
230 Calories

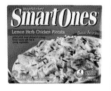

SMART ONES
Lemon Herb Chicken
Piccata
1 meal
230 Calories

DINNER SIDES

Build-a-Meal
250-Calorie Dinner Sides

Low Carb= **Sodium Controlled=** **Vegetarian=**

AMY'S
Refried Black Beans
½ can
245 Calories

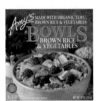

AMY'S
Brown Rice &
Vegetable Bowl
1 bowl
260 Calories

AMY'S
Pasta & 3 Bean Soup
1 can
260 Calories

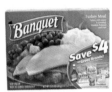

BANQUET
Turkey Meal
1 meal
250 Calories

BARBER FOODS
Cordon Bleu Stuffed
Chicken Breasts
1 piece
250 Calories

CAMPBELL'S
Old Fashioned Vegetable
Beef Chunky Soup
1 can
240 Calories

CAMPBELL'S
Cream of Broccoli
Condensed Soup
1 can
250 Calories

CAMPBELL'S
Vegetable
Condensed Soup
1 can
250 Calories

DOLE
Creamy Coleslaw Kit
1 bag
241 Calories

DR. PRAEGER'S
Meatless All American
Burger
2 burgers
260 Calories

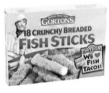

GORTON'S
Crunchy Breaded
Fish Sticks
6 pieces
250 Calories

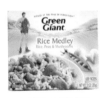

GREEN GIANT
Rice Medley
1 package
250 Calories

Build-a-Meal
250-Calorie Dinner Sides

Low Carb= 🍞 **Sodium Controlled=** 🧂 **Vegetarian=** 🥕

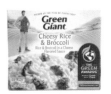

GREEN GIANT
Cheesy Rice & Broccoli
1 package
270 Calories
🥕

HEALTHY CHOICE
Steaming Entrées
Roasted Chicken Verde
1 meal
240 Calories
🧂

HEALTHY CHOICE
Café Steamers Lemon
Garlic Chicken & Shrimp
1 meal
260 Calories
🧂

HEALTHY CHOICE
Café Steamers Grilled
Chicken Marinara
1 meal
260 Calories
🧂

HEALTHY CHOICE
All Natural Portabella
Spinach Parmesan
1 meal
270 Calories
🧂 🥕

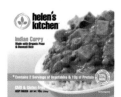

HELEN'S KITCHEN
Indian Curry
1 container
260 Calories
🧂 🥕

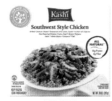

KASHI
Southwest Style Chicken
1 meal
240 Calories

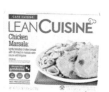

LEAN CUISINE
Cafe Cuisine
Chicken Marsala
1 meal
250 Calories

LEAN CUISINE
Comfort Cuisine
Baked Chicken
1 meal
250 Calories
🧂

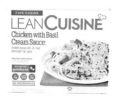

LEAN CUISINE
Cafe Cuisine Chicken with
Basil Cream Sauce
1 meal
250 Calories
🧂

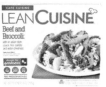

LEAN CUISINE
Cafe Cuisine Beef
and Broccoli
1 meal
260 Calories
🧂

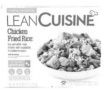

LEAN CUISINE
Simple Favorites Chicken
Fried Rice
1 meal
260 Calories
🧂

DINNER SIDES

161

Build-a-Meal
250-Calorie Dinner Sides

Low Carb= 🍞 **Sodium Controlled=** 🧂 **Vegetarian=** 🌿

LEAN CUISINE
Market Creations
Garlic Chicken
1 meal
270 Calories

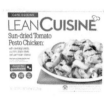

LEAN CUISINE
Cafe Cuisine Sun-Dried
Tomato Pesto Chicken
1 meal
270 Calories
🧂

LEAN POCKETS
Whole Grain Chicken
Broccoli and Cheddar
1 piece
250 Calories
🧂

LEAN POCKETS
Whole Grain Ham
& Cheddar
1 piece
270 Calories

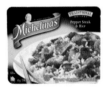

MICHELINA'S
Traditional Recipes Pep-
per Steak & Rice
1 meal
260 Calories

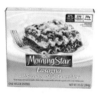

MORNINGSTAR FARMS
Lasagna with Sausage
Style Crumbles
1 meal
270 Calories
🧂 🌿

SIMPLY ASIA
Sesame Chicken Soup
Bowl
1 bowl
250 Calories

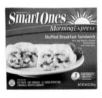

SMART ONES
Morning Express Stuffed
Breakfast Sandwich
1 meal
240 Calories

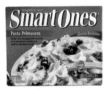

SMART ONES
Pasta Primavera
1 meal
250 Calories
🌿

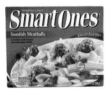

SMART ONES
Swedish Meatballs
1 meal
270 Calories

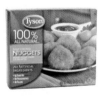

TYSON
100% Natural Nuggets
6 pieces
270 Calories
🍞

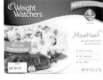

WEIGHT WATCHERS
Meatloaf
1 meal
240 Calories

ALL-AMERICAN DIET

Build-a-Meal
300-Calorie Dinner Sides

Low Carb= 🍞 **Sodium Controlled=** 🧂 **Vegetarian=** 🌱

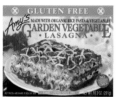

AMY'S
Gluten Free Garden Vegetable Lasagna
1 container
290 Calories
🌱

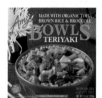

AMY'S
Teriyaki Bowl
1 bowl
290 Calories
🌱

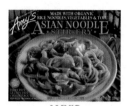

AMY'S
Asian Noodle Stir-Fry
1 container
300 Calories
🌱

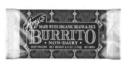

AMY'S
Non-Dairy Bean & Rice Burrito
1 burrito
300 Calories
🌱

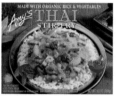

AMY'S
Thai Stir-Fry
1 package
310 Calories
🧂 🌱

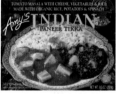

AMY'S
Indian Paneer Tikka
1 meal
320 Calories
🌱

AMY'S
Tuscan Bean & Rice Soup
1 can
320 Calories
🧂 🌱

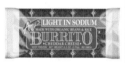

AMY'S
Light in Sodium Cheddar Burrito
1 burrito
330 Calories
🌱

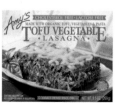

AMY'S
Tofu Vegetable Lasagna
1 container
330 Calories
🌱

ANNIE CHUN'S
Organic Chicken and Vegetable Potstickers
1 container
330 Calories

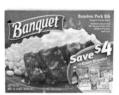

BANQUET
Boneless Pork Rib
1 meal
320 Calories

BETTY CROCKER
Roasted Garlic Instant Potatoes
1 package
320 Calories

Build-a-Meal
300-Calorie Dinner Sides

Low Carb= **Sodium Controlled=** **Vegetarian=**

BIRDS EYE
Vegetables & Shells in
Garlic Butter Sauce
1 package
270 Calories

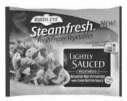

BIRDS EYE
Lightly Sauced Vegetables
Roasted Red Potatoes
with Chive Butter Sauce
1 bag
280 Calories

BIRDS EYE
Steamfresh Long Grain
White Rice
1 bag
320 Calories

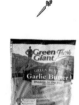

CAMPBELL'S
Grilled Sirloin Burger
with Hearty Vegetables
Chunky Soup
1 bowl
280 Calories

CAMPBELL'S
Creamy Chicken Noodle
Condensed Soup
1 can
300 Calories

CAMPBELL'S
Creamy Chicken & Dump-
lings Chunky Soup
1 can
320 Calories

CAMPBELL'S
Tomato Bisque Con-
densed Soup
1 can
325 Calories

CEDARLANE
Low Fat Garden Veg-
etable Enchiladas
1 package
280 Calories

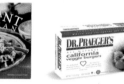

CEDARLANE
Eggplant Parmesan
1 package
320 Calories

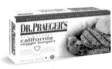

DR. PRAEGER'S
California Veggie Burgers
3 burgers
330 Calories

FRESH EXPRESS
House Ranch Salad Kit
1 package
300 Calories

GREEN GIANT
Green Beans & Garlic
Butter
1 bag
330 Calories

Build-a-Meal
300-Calorie Dinner Sides

Low Carb= **Sodium Controlled=** **Vegetarian=**

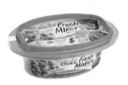

HEALTHY CHOICE
Fresh Mixers Penne &
Roasted Red Pepper
Alfredo
1 package
290 Calories

HEALTHY CHOICE
Chicken & Dumplings
Soup
1 can
300 Calories

HEALTHY CHOICE
Café Steamers Chicken
Pesto Classico
1 meal
310 Calories

HEALTHY CHOICE
Split Pea & Ham Soup
1 can
320 Calories

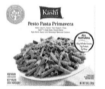

KASHI
Pesto Pasta Primavera
1 container
290 Calories

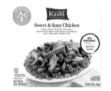

KASHI
Sweet & Sour Chicken
1 container
320 Calories

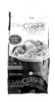

LEAN CUISINE
Market Creations Sweet
and Spicy Ginger Chicken
1 meal
280 Calories

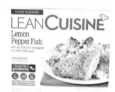

LEAN CUISINE
Cafe Cuisine Lemon Pepper Fish
1 meal
290 Calories

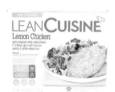

LEAN CUISINE
Spa Cuisine Lemon
Chicken
1 meal
290 Calories

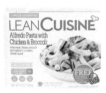

LEAN CUISINE
Simple Favorites Alfredo
Pasta with Chicken
& Broccoli
1 meal
300 Calories

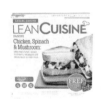

LEAN CUISINE
Casual Cuisine Chicken
Spinach Mushroom Panini
1 panini
310 Calories

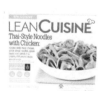

LEAN CUISINE
Spa Cuisine Thai Style
Noodles with Chicken
1 meal
310 Calories

Build-a-Meal
300-Calorie Dinner Sides

Low Carb= 🍞 **Sodium Controlled=** 🧂 **Vegetarian=** 🌿

LEAN CUISINE
Casual Cuisine Spinach,
Artichoke & Chicken
Panini
1 panini
320 Calories

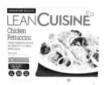

LEAN CUISINE
Dinnertime Selects
Chicken Fettuccini
1 meal
330 Calories

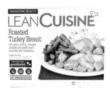

LEAN CUISINE
Dinnertime Selects
Roasted Turkey Breast
1 meal
290 Calories

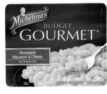

MICHELINA'S
Budget Gourmet Home-
style Macaroni & Cheese
1 package
280 Calories

🌿

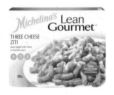

MICHELINA'S
Lean Gourmet Three
Cheese Ziti Marinara
1 package
300 Calories

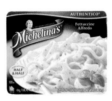

MICHELINA'S
Authentico Fettucine
Alfredo
1 package
330 Calories

READY PAC
Spinach Dijon Bistro
Salad
1 package
280 Calories

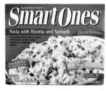

SMART ONES
Pasta with Ricotta and
Spinach
1 meal
280 Calories

🌿

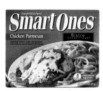

SMART ONES
Chicken Parmesan
1 meal
290 Calories

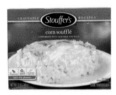

STOUFFER'S
Craveable Recipes Corn
Soufflé
1 meal
300 Calories

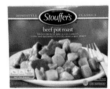

STOUFFER'S
Homestyle Classics Beef
Pot Roast
1 meal
320 Calories

ALL-AMERICAN DIET

Build-a-Meal
10- to 50-Calorie Fruits and Vegetables

Low Carb= **Sodium Controlled=** **Vegetarian=**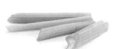

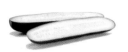

CUCUMBER
1 medium
8 Calories

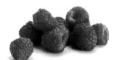

RASPBERRIES
10 berries
10 Calories

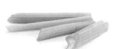

CELERY
4 5" stalks
12 Calories

**EARTHBOUND FARMS
ORGANIC**
Baby Spinach
1 5-ounce package
17 Calories

FRESH EXPRESS
Sweet Butter
1 package
20 Calories

FRESH EXPRESS
50/50 Mix
1 package
20 Calories

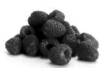

RASPBERRIES
20 berries
20 Calories

TOMATO
1 medium
22 Calories

GREEN PEPPER
1 medium
24 Calories

READY PAC
Fresh European Style
Lafayette
1 bag
25 Calories

**EARTHBOUND FARMS
ORGANIC**
Baby Romaine
1 5-ounce package
26 Calories

**EARTHBOUND FARMS
ORGANIC**
Mixed Baby Greens
1 5-ounce package
26 Calories

Build-a-Meal
10- to 50-Calorie Fruits and Vegetables

Low Carb= Sodium Controlled=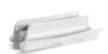 Vegetarian=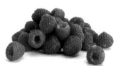

FRESH EXPRESS
Italian
1 package
30 Calories

READY PAC
Fresh European Style
Spring Mix
1 bag
30 Calories

RASPBERRIES
30 berries
30 Calories

CELERY
5 8" stalks
30 Calories

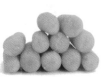

BABY CARROTS
11 carrots
30 Calories

RED PEPPER
1 medium
31 Calories

EARTHBOUND FARMS ORGANIC
Baby Arugula
1 5-ounce package
34 Calories

CLEMENTINE
1 fruit
35 Calories

GRAPEFRUIT
½ fruit (3¾" diameter)
37 Calories

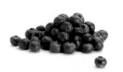

READY PAC
Fresh European Style
Santa Barbara
1 7-ounce bag
38 Calories

BLUEBERRIES
50 berries
39 Calories

DOLE
7 Lettuces
1 bag
40 Calories

ALL-AMERICAN DIET

Build-a-Meal
10- to 50-Calorie Fruits and Vegetables

Low Carb= **Sodium Controlled=** **Vegetarian=**

FRESH EXPRESS
Baby Spinach
1 package
40 Calories

READY PAC
Spinach
1 bag
40 Calories

TAYLOR ORGANIC
Baby Spring Mix
1 5-ounce package
40 Calories

FRESH EXPRESS
5-Lettuce Mix
1 package
45 Calories

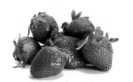

STRAWBERRIES
8 large berries
(1⅜" diameter)
46 Calories

YELLOW PEPPER
1 large
50 Calories

Build-a-Meal
51- to 100-Calorie Fruits and Vegetables

Low Carb= **Sodium Controlled=** **Vegetarian=**

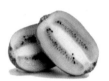

KIWI
1 fruit
52 Calories

MOTT'S
Sliced Apples
1 bag
57 Calories

DEL MONTE
Fresh Cut Leaf Spinach
1 7.75-ounce can
60 Calories

FRESH EXPRESS
American Mix
1 package
60 Calories

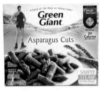

GREEN GIANT
Asparagus Cuts
1 box
60 Calories

ARTICHOKE
1 medium
60 Calories

BLACKBERRIES
1 cup or ½ pint
62 Calories

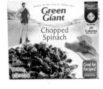

GREEN GIANT
Chopped Spinach
1 box
63 Calories

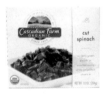

CASCADIAN FARM
Cut Spinach
1 box
66 Calories

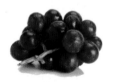

RED GRAPES
20 grapes
66 Calories

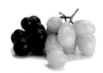

RED & GREEN GRAPES
20 grapes
66 Calories

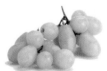

GREEN GRAPES
20 grapes
66 Calories

Build-a-Meal
50- to 100-Calorie Fruits and Vegetables

Low Carb= **Sodium Controlled=** **Vegetarian=**

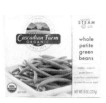

CASCADIAN FARM
Whole Petite Green Beans
1 box
68 Calories

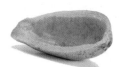

PAPAYA
½ medium
68 Calories

NAVEL ORANGE
1 fruit
69 Calories

DEL MONTE
Fresh Cut Sliced Beets
1 8.25-ounce can
70 Calories

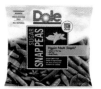

DOLE
Sugar Snap Peas
½ package
70 Calories

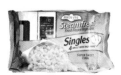

BIRDS EYE
Steamfresh Singles Super
Sweet Corn
1 single bag
80 Calories

DEL MONTE
Mixed Vegetables
1 8.25-ounce can
80 Calories

GREEN GIANT
Broccoli Florettes
1 package
80 Calories

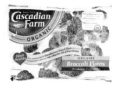

CASCADIAN FARM
Organic Broccoli Florets
1 10-ounce bag
84 Calories

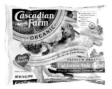

CASCADIAN FARM
Premium Organic
California Style Blend
1 10-ounce bag
85 Calories

GREEN GIANT
Stringless Sugar
Snap Peas
½ package
88 Calories

MELISSA'S
Baby Beets
1 package
91 Calories

Build-a-Meal
51- to 100-Calorie Fruits and Vegetables

Low Carb= **Sodium Controlled=** **Vegetarian=**

GREEN APPLE
1 medium
95 Calories

RED APPLE
1 medium
95 Calories

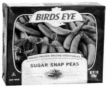

BIRDS EYE
Sugar Snap Peas
1 package
100 Calories

DOLE
Broccoli & Cauliflower
1 package
100 Calories

Build-a-Meal
101- to 280-Calorie Fruits and Vegetables

Low Carb= **Sodium Controlled=** 🧂 **Vegetarian=** 🌿

PEAR
1 medium
103 Calories

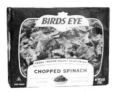

BIRDS EYE
Chopped Spinach
1 package
105 Calories

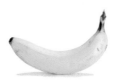

BANANA
1 medium
105 Calories

DEL MONTE
Specialties Peas & Carrots
1 8.5-ounce can
110 Calories

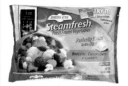

BIRDS EYE
Steamfresh Broccoli Cauliflower and Carrots
1 bag
120 Calories

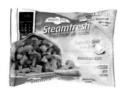

BIRDS EYE
Steamfresh Broccoli Cuts
1 bag
120 Calories

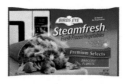

BIRDS EYE
Steamfresh Premium Selects Broccoli Florets
1 bag
120 Calories

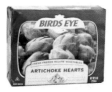

BIRDS EYE
Artichoke Hearts
1 package
120 Calories

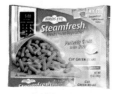

BIRDS EYE
Steamfresh Cut Green Beans
1 package
120 Calories

DEL MONTE
Fresh Cut Whole Kernel Corn
1 8.75-ounce can
120 Calories

DOLE
Broccoli & Carrots
1 package
120 Calories

DOLE
Broccoli Florets
1 package
120 Calories

Build-a-Meal
101- to 280-Calorie Fruits and Vegetables

Low Carb= **Sodium Controlled=** 🧂 **Vegetarian=** 🌱

DOLE
Stir Fry Medley
1 package
120 Calories

DOLE
Vegetable Medley
1 package
120 Calories

GREEN GIANT
Vegetable Medley
1 package
120 Calories

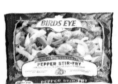

BIRDS EYE
Pepper Stir-Fry
1 bag
125 Calories

GREEN GIANT
Steamers Sugar Snap
Peas
1 package
135 Calories

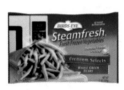

BIRDS EYE
Steamfresh Premium Se-
lects Whole Green Beans
1 package
140 Calories

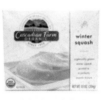

CASCADIAN FARM
Winter Squash
1 box
140 Calories

AVOCADO
½ fruit
156 Calories

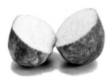

POTATO
1 medium
168 Calories

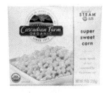

CASCADIAN FARM
Super Sweet Corn
1 box
180 Calories

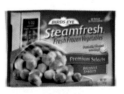

BIRDS EYE
Steamfresh Premium Se-
lects Brussels Sprouts
1 bag
180 Calories

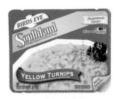

BIRDS EYE
Southland Yellow Turnips
1 package
210 Calories

ALL-AMERICAN DIET

Build-a-Meal
101- to 280-Calorie Fruits and Vegetables

Low Carb= Sodium Controlled= Vegetarian=

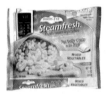

BIRDS EYE

Steamfresh Mixed
Vegetables
1 bag
240 Calories

GREEN GIANT

Steamers Baby Sweet
Peas
1 box
240 Calories

CASCADIAN FARM

Sweet Peas
1 10-ounce bag
245 Calories

CASCADIAN FARM

Sweet Corn
1 10-ounce bag
270 Calories

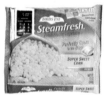

BIRDS EYE

Super Sweet Corn
1 bag
280 Calories

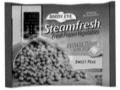

BIRDS EYE

Steamfresh Sweet Peas
1 bag
280 Calories

Condiments

Condiments are counted as sides. As you can see, there are more condiments than those pictured here, and you can definitely stray from this list. The biggest difficulty with condiments is finding single-serving units. If you can't find them, be sure to follow these guidelines to ensure that you don't accidentally rack up calories.

- Premeasure *all* condiments with measuring spoons, following the serving size indicated on the nutrition label.
- Use a fork to drizzle salad dressing on your salads—don't just dump it on.
- Always use less than you think you need—a little can go a long way!
- Go for low-calorie and/or fat-free options.

Build-a-Meal
Condiments

Low Carb= Sodium Controlled= Vegetarian=

DOMINO
Sugar Packets
1 packet
15 Calories

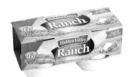

HIDDEN VALLEY RANCH
Single Cups
1 cup
200 Calories

I CAN'T BELIEVE IT'S NOT BUTTER
Original Spray
1 spray
0 Calories

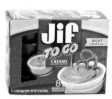

JIF
To Go Creamy Peanut Butter Singles
1 single cup
250 Calories

JUSTIN'S
Honey Peanut Butter
1 packet
190 Calories

JUSTIN'S
Classic Almond Butter
1 packet
200 Calories

JUSTIN'S
Classic Peanut Butter
1 packet
200 Calories

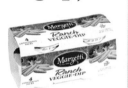

MARZETTI
Ranch Veggie-Dip Convenience Packs
1 3-ounce cup
360 Calories

NESTLÉ
Coffee-mate Original
1 packet
15 Calories

NESTLÉ
Coffee-mate French Vanilla
1 packet
60 Calories

PHILADELPHIA
Regular Cream Cheese Spread Minis
1 mini
100 Calories

PHILADELPHIA
Regular Chive & Onion Minis
1 mini
100 Calories

Build-a-Meal
Condiments

Low Carb= **Sodium Controlled=** **Vegetarian=**

WISH-BONE
Salad Spritzers Italian
Vinaigrette Dressing
10 sprays
10 Calories

WISH-BONE
Salad Spritzers Balsamic
Breeze Vinaigrette
Dressing
10 sprays
10 Calories

WISH-BONE
Salad Spritzers Ranch
Vinaigrette Dressing
10 sprays
15 Calories

Build-a-Meal
50-Calorie Desserts

Low Carb= 🍞 **Sodium Controlled=** 🧂 **Vegetarian=** 🥕

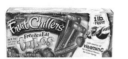
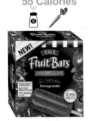

DEL MONTE
Fruit Chillers Freeze & Eat
Tubes, Strawberry Snow
Storm
1 tube
55 Calories
🧂 🥕

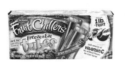
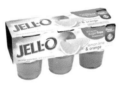

DEL MONTE
Fruit Chillers Freeze &
Eat Tubes, Grape Berry
Blizzard
1 tube
55 Calories
🧂 🥕

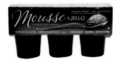

DREYER'S/EDY'S
Strawberry, Tangerine,
Raspberry No Sugar
Added Fruit Bars
1 bar
30 Calories
🧂 🥕

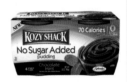

DREYER'S/EDY'S
Lime, Strawberry, Wild
Berry Fruit Bars
1 bar
45 Calories
🧂 🥕

DREYER'S/EDY'S
Pomegranate Antioxidant
Fruit Bars
1 bar
70 Calories
🧂 🥕

JELL-O
10 Calories Sugar Free
Lemon-Lime and Orange
1 container
10 Calories
🍞 🧂 🥕

JELL-O
Mousse Temptations
Chocolate Indulgence
1 container
60 Calories
🍞 🧂 🥕

KOZY SHACK
No Sugar Added
Pudding, Chocolate Mint
1 snack cup
70 Calories
🍞 🧂 🥕

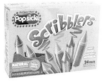

POPSICLE
Scribblers
1 pop
30 Calories
🧂 🥕

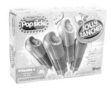

POPSICLE
Ice Pops, Jolly Rancher
1 pop
45 Calories
🧂 🥕

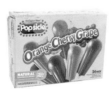

POPSICLE
Ice Pops, Orange Cherry
Grape
1 pop
45 Calories
🧂 🥕

**STRETCH ISLAND
FRUIT CO.**
All-Natural Fruit Strip,
Autumn Apple
1 strip
70 Calories
🧂 🥕

Build-a-Meal
100-Calorie Desserts

Low Carb= **Sodium Controlled=** **Vegetarian=**

DREYER'S/EDY'S
Grape Fruit Bars
1 bar
80 Calories

DREYER'S/EDY'S
Lemonade Fruit Bars
1 bar
80 Calories

DREYER'S/EDY'S
Strawberry Fruit Bars
1 bar
80 Calories

DREYER'S/EDY'S
Lime Fruit Bars
1 bar
80 Calories

DREYER'S/EDY'S
Tangerine Fruit Bars
1 bar
80 Calories

DREYER'S/EDY'S
Creamy Coconut Fruit
Bars
1 bar
120 Calories

HOSTESS
100 Calorie Packs Chocolate Cake with Creamy
Filling
1 package
100 Calories

HOSTESS
100 Calorie Packs Cinnamon Streusel Coffee Cakes
1 package
100 Calories

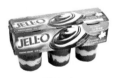

JELL-O
100 Calorie Fat Free
Chocolate Vanilla Swirls
1 container
100 Calories

KEEBLER
100 Calorie Right Bites
Mini Fudge Stripes
1 pouch
100 Calories

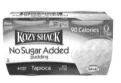

KOZY SHACK
No Sugar Added
Pudding, Tapioca
1 snack cup
90 Calories

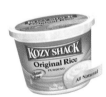

KOZY SHACK
Original Rice Pudding
1 snack cup
90 Calories

ALL-AMERICAN DIET

Build-a-Meal
100-Calorie Desserts

Low Carb= Sodium Controlled= Vegetarian=

NABISCO
100 Cal Variety Pack
(Oreo, Chips Ahoy,
Lorna Doone)
1 pouch
100 Calories

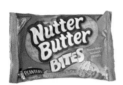

NABISCO
Nutter Butter Bites
1 1-ounce bag
130 Calories

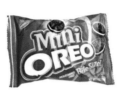

NABISCO
Mini Oreo Cookies
1 1-ounce bag
130 Calories

PEPPERIDGE FARM
Milano Cookies 2-pack
1 package
120 Calories

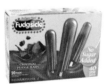

POPSICLE
Original Fudgsicle No
Sugar Added
1 pop
80 Calories

SKINNY COW
Caramel Truffle Low Fat
Ice Cream Bars
1 bar
100 Calories

SKINNY COW
Chocolate Truffle Low Fat
Ice Cream Bars
1 bar
100 Calories

SKINNY COW
French Vanilla Truffle Low
Fat Ice Cream Bars
1 bar
100 Calories

SKINNY COW
Low Fat Fudge Bar
1 bar
100 Calories

SNACK PACK
Fat Free Tapioca
1 cup
80 Calories

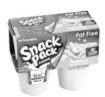

SNACK PACK
Fat Free Chocolate
1 cup
80 Calories

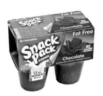

WEIGHT WATCHERS
Giant Chocolate Cookies
& Cream Ice Cream Bars
1 bar
130 Calories

DESSERTS

Build-a-Meal
100-Calorie Desserts

Low Carb= 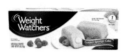 **Sodium Controlled=** **Vegetarian=**

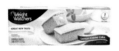

WEIGHT WATCHERS
Lemon Créme Cake
1 cake
80 calories

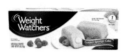

WEIGHT WATCHERS
Golden Sponge Cake with
Creamy Filling
1 cake
80 calories

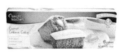

WEIGHT WATCHERS
Carrot Crème Cake
1 cake
90 Calories

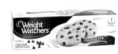

WEIGHT WATCHERS
Chocolate Chip Cookies
1 cookie
90 calories

WEIGHT WATCHERS
English Toffee Crunch Ice
Cream Bars
1 bar
100 Calories

WEIGHT WATCHERS
Vanilla Ice Cream
Sandwiches (rectangular
bars)
1 sandwich
120 Calories

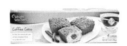

WEIGHT WATCHERS
Coffee Cake
1 cake
120 Calories

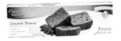

WEIGHT WATCHERS
Chocolate Brownie
1 brownie
130 Calories

Build-a-Meal
150-Calorie Desserts

Low Carb=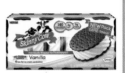 Sodium Controlled=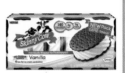 Vegetarian=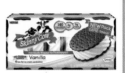

ENTENMANN'S
Mini Cakes Pound Cake
1 cake
170 Calories

HERSHEY'S
York Peppermint Pattie
1 1.4-ounce patty
140 Calories

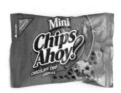

NABISCO
Mini Chips Ahoy
1 1-ounce bag
140 Calories

SKINNY COW
No Sugar Added Vanilla
Low Fat Ice Cream
Sandwiches
1 sandwich
140 Calories

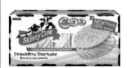

SKINNY COW
Strawberry Shortcake
Low Fat Ice Cream
Sandwiches
1 sandwich
140 Calories

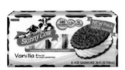

SKINNY COW
Vanilla Low Fat Ice Cream
Sandwiches
1 sandwich
140 Calories

SKINNY COW
Chocolate with Fudge
Low Fat Ice Cream Cones
1 cone
150 Calories

SKINNY COW
Chocolate Fudge Brownie
Low Fat Ice Cream
1 5.8-ounce container
150 Calories

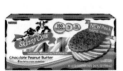

SKINNY COW
Chocolate Peanut Butter
Low Fat Ice Cream
Sandwiches
1 sandwich
150 Calories

SKINNY COW
Cookies 'n Cream Low
Fat Ice Cream
1 5.8-ounce container
150 Calories

SKINNY COW
Dulce de Leche Low Fat
Ice Cream
1 5.8-ounce container
150 Calories

SKINNY COW
Mint with Fudge Low Fat
Ice Cream Cones
1 cone
150 Calories

Build-a-Meal
150-Calorie Desserts

Low Carb= **Sodium Controlled=** **Vegetarian=**

SKINNY COW
Low Fat Strawberry
Cheesecake Ice Cream
1 5.8-ounce container
150 Calories

SKINNY COW
Vanilla with Caramel Low
Fat Ice Cream Cones
1 cone
150 Calories

SKINNY COW
Caramel Cone Low Fat
Ice Cream
1 5.8-ounce container
170 Calories

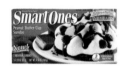

SMART ONES
Peanut Butter Cup
Sundae
1 sundae
170 Calories

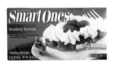

SMART ONES
Strawberry Shortcake
1 cake
170 Calories

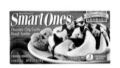

SMART ONES
Chocolate Chip Cookie
Dough Sundae
1 sundae
170 Calories

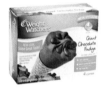

WEIGHT WATCHERS
Giant Chocolate Fudge
Ice Cream Sundae Cones
1 cone
140 Calories

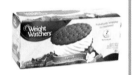

WEIGHT WATCHERS
Vanilla Ice Cream
Sandwiches
1 sandwich
140 Calories

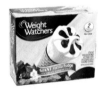

WEIGHT WATCHERS
Giant Vanilla Fudge
Sundae Cones
1 cone
140 Calories

WEIGHT WATCHERS
Mint Chocolate Chip Ice
Cream Cups
1 cup
140 Calories

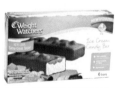

WEIGHT WATCHERS
Ice Cream Candy Bars
1 bar
150 Calories

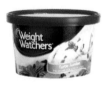

WEIGHT WATCHERS
Turtle Sundae Ice Cream
Cups
1 cup
170 Calories

ALL-AMERICAN DIET

Build-a-Meal
200-Calorie Desserts

Low Carb= Sodium Controlled= Vegetarian=

ENTENMANN'S
Mini Cakes, Chocolate Chip
1 cake
190 Calories

HÄAGEN-DAZS
Single Serve Vanilla
1 container
220 Calories

HÄAGEN-DAZS
Single Serve Strawberry
1 container
220 Calories

HOSTESS
100 Calorie Packs Strawberry w/Cream Cheese Icing and Creamy Filling
2 packages
200 Calories

KEEBLER
100 Calorie Right Bites
Fudge Dipped Pretzels
2 pouches
200 Calories

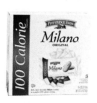

PEPPERIDGE FARM
100 Calorie Pouches
Milano Cookies
2 pouches
200 Calories

SKINNY COW
White Mint Truffle Low Fat
Ice Cream Bars
2 bars
200 Calories

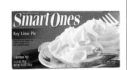

SMART ONES
Key Lime Pie
1 pie
190 Calories

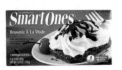

SMART ONES
Brownie À La Mode
1 piece
200 Calories

TWIX
Mini Ice Cream Bars
2 bars
180 Calories

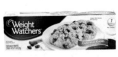

WEIGHT WATCHERS
Oatmeal Raisin Cookies
2 cookies
200 Calories

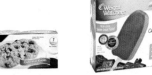

WEIGHT WATCHERS
Giant Chocolate Fudge
Ice Cream Bars
2 bars
220 Calories

DESSERTS

185

Build-a-Meal
25-Calorie Beverages

Low Carb= Sodium Controlled= Vegetarian=

BEVERAGES

CAMPBELL'S
V8 100% Vegetable Juice
1 5.5-ounce can
30 Calories

CAMPBELL'S
V8 Low Sodium
Vegetable Juice
1 5.5-ounce can
30 Calories

CAPRI SUN
Roarin' Waters,
Tropical Fruit
1 pouch
35 Calories

HINT
Unsweetened Essence
Water. Strawberry-Kiwi
1 bottle
0 Calories

HONEST TEA
Organic Passion Fruit
Green Tea
1 16-ounce bottle
0 Calories

HONEST TEA
Just Black Tea
1 16-ounce bottle
0 Calories

HONEST TEA
Just Green Tea
1 16-ounce bottle
0 Calories

HONEST TEA
Community Green Tea
1 16-ounce bottle
34 Calories

HONEST TEA
Moroccan Mint Green Tea
1 16-ounce bottle
34 Calories

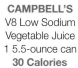

KOOL-AID
On the Go Tropical Punch
1 packet
5 Calories

LIPTON
Lemon Iced Tea on the
Go Packets
1 packet
0 Calories

PEPSI
Sprite Zero
1 can
0 Calories

Build-a-Meal
25-Calorie Beverages

Low Carb= **Sodium Controlled=** **Vegetarian=**

PEPSI
Diet Pepsi
1 can
0 Calories

RED BULL
Sugarfree Energy Shot
1 2-oz. bottle
2 Calories

RED BULL
Energy Shot
1 2-ounce bottle
25 Calories

SNAPPLE
Diet Peach or Green
1 16-ounce bottle
0 Calories

SNAPPLE
Diet Peach Tea
1 16-ounce bottle
0 Calories

VITAMIN WATER
Zero Go-Go
1 16-ounce. bottle
0 Calories

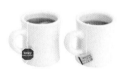

HOT TEA
1 mug
0 Calories

WATER
1 glass
0 Calories

WATER
1 bottle
0 Calories

BLACK COFFEE
1 mug
5 Calories

Build-a-Meal
50-Calorie Beverages

Low Carb= **Sodium Controlled=** **Vegetarian=**

APPLE & EVE
Big Bird's Apple
1 box
55 Calories

HONEST KIDS
Super Fruit Punch
1 pouch
40 Calories

HONEST KIDS
Appley Ever After
1 pouch
40 Calories

HONEST KIDS
Berry Berry Good Lemonade
1 pouch
40 Calories

HONEST TEA
Lori's Lemon Tea
1 16-ounce bottle
60 Calories

HONEST TEA
Peach Oo-La-Long
1 16-ounce bottle
60 Calories

ZICO
Pure Premium Coconut
Water, Pomberry
1 14-ounce bottle
60 Calories

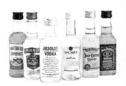

LIQUOR
1 mini bottle
60 Calories

BEVERAGES

Build-a-Meal
75-Calorie Beverages

Low Carb= 🍞 **Sodium Controlled=** 🧂 **Vegetarian=** 🌱

APPLE & EVE
Elmo's Punch
1 box
65 Calories
🧂 🌱

APPLE & EVE
Fruitables Berry Berry
1 box
70 Calories
🧂 🌱

APPLE & EVE
Fruitables Tropical Orange
1 box
70 Calories
🧂 🌱

CAMPBELL'S
Tomato Juice from
Concentrate
12-fl.ounce bottle
75 Calories
🧂 🌱

HONEST MATE
Maqui Berry Mate
1 16-ounce bottle
70 Calories
🧂 🌱

HONEST MATE
Sublime Mate
1 16-ounce bottle
70 Calories
🧂 🌱

HONEST TEA
Caffeine-Free
Pomegranate Red Tea
1 16-ounce bottle
70 Calories
🧂 🌱

HONEST TEA
Mango Açaí White Tea
1 16-ounce bottle
70 Calories
🧂 🌱

HONEST TEA
Organic Honey Green Tea
1 16-ounce bottle
74 Calories
🧂 🌱

HONEST TEA
Organic Lemon Black Tea
1 16-ounce bottle
85 Calories
🧂 🌱

HONEST TEA
Organic Pomegranate
White Tea
1 16-ounce bottle
85 Calories
🧂 🌱

KOOL-AID
Jammers Tropical Punch
1 pouch
70 Calories
🧂 🌱

Build-a-Meal
100-Calorie Beverages

Low Carb= **Sodium Controlled=** **Vegetarian=**

HI-C
Orange Lava Burst
1 box
90 Calories

HI-C
Grabbin' Grape
1 box
90 Calories

HI-C
Flashin' Fruit Punch
1 box
90 Calories

HONEST ADE
Superfruit Punch
1 16-ounce bottle
100 Calories

HONEST TEA
Limeade
1 16-ounce bottle
100 Calories

HONEST TEA
Organic Half Tea & Half
Lemonade
1 16-ounce bottle
100 Calories

HORIZON ORGANIC
Lowfat Milk
1 8-ounce box
110 Calories

JUICY JUICE
Apple
1 6.75-ounce box
100 Calories

JUICY JUICE
Punch
1 6.75-ounce box
100 Calories

JUICY JUICE
Grape
1 6.75-ounce box
100 Calories

JUICY JUICE
Berry
1 6.75-ounce box
100 Calories

JUICY JUICE
Orange Tangerine
1 6.75-ounce box
100 Calories

Build-a-Meal
100-Calorie Beverages

Low Carb= **Sodium Controlled=** **Vegetarian=**

MINUTE MAID
Apple Juice
1 6.75-ounce box
100 Calories

MINUTE MAID
Fruit Punch
1 6.75-ounce box
100 Calories

MINUTE MAID
Apple White Grape Juice
1 6.75-ounce box
100 Calories

NEWMAN'S OWN
Virgin Lemon Aided
Iced Tea
1 6.75-ounce box
100 Calories

NEWMAN'S OWN
Virgin Lemonade
1 6.75-ounce box
100 Calories

ORGANIC VALLEY
1% Lowfat Milk
1 8-ounce box
110 Calories

TROPICANA
Pure Premium Orange
Juice
1 8-ounce box
110 Calories

VITAMIN WATER
Revive
1 16-ounce bottle
100 Calories

ALL-AMERICAN DIET

Build-a-Meal
150-Calorie Beverages

Low Carb= **Sodium Controlled=** **Vegetarian=**

ARIZONA TEA
Half and Half Iced Tea
Lemonade
1 24-ounce can
150 Calories

BOLTHOUSE FARMS
Carrot Juice
1 14.5-ounce bottle
140 Calories

HORIZON ORGANIC
Lowfat Chocolate Milk
1 8-ounce box
150 Calories

ORGANIC VALLEY
1% Lowfat Chocolate Milk
1 8-ounce box
150 Calories

ORGANIC VALLEY
1% Lowfat Vanilla Milk
1 8-ounce box
150 Calories

Restaurant Foods

(Listed by restaurant name with options from lowest to highest calorie content)

Are you at a restaurant or fast-food outlet and don't see your particular food choice listed on these pages? That's because we tried to pick foods that are healthier options. However, that's not to say that you can't have it if it fits into your calorie level for your specific meal plan. Always keep in mind, these meal plans are not meant to be followed precisely, and there is a "fudge factor" of 10 to 20 calories per day—but that goes both ways. If you go over your calorie limit by 20 calories today, try to go under your limit by 20 calories tomorrow.

Build-a-Meal
7-Eleven

Low Carb= **Sodium Controlled=** **Vegetarian=**

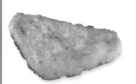

7-ELEVEN
Hashbrowns
1 piece
100 Calories

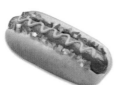

7-ELEVEN
Big Bite
1 hot dog
180 Calories

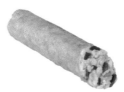

7-ELEVEN
Bacon, Egg, Cheese and
Potato Taquito
1 taquito
190 Calories

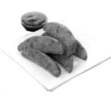

7-ELEVEN
Potato Wedges
6 pieces
240 Calories

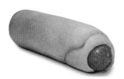

7-ELEVEN
Corn Dog Roller
1 hot dog
320 Calories

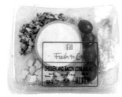

7-ELEVEN
Fresh to Go Chicken and
Bacon Cobb Salad
1 container
350 Calories

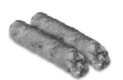

7-ELEVEN
Buffalo Chicken Taquitos
2 taquitos
360 Calories

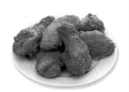

7-ELEVEN
Wings
6 pieces
360 Calories

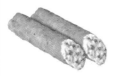

7-ELEVEN
Jalapeño Cream Cheese
Taquitos
2 taquitos
480 Calories

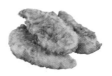

7-ELEVEN
Chicken Tenders
3 pieces
480 Calories

RESTAURANTS

Build-a-Meal
Applebee's

Low Carb= 🍞 **Sodium Controlled=** 🧂 **Vegetarian=** 🌿

APPLEBEE'S
Seasonal Veggies
1 order
50 Calories
🧂 🌿

APPLEBEE'S
Side Caesar Salad
1 order
310 Calories
🍞 🌿

APPLEBEE'S
Weight Watchers Spicy
Pineapple Glazed Shrimp
and Spinach
1 order
310 Calories

APPLEBEE'S
House Salad
1 Order with Mexi-Ranch
Dressing
320 Calories
🍞 🌿

APPLEBEE'S
Weight Watchers Paradise
Chicken Salad
1 order
340 Calories

APPLEBEE'S
Weight Watchers Cajun
Lime Tilapia
1 order
350 Calories

APPLEBEE'S
Grilled Shrimp
and Island Rice
1 order
370 Calories

APPLEBEE'S
Weight Watchers Steak
and Potato Salad
1 order
380 Calories

APPLEBEE'S
Asiago Peppercorn
Steak with Sides
1 order
390 Calories
🍞

APPLEBEE'S
Half Grilled Chicken
Caesar Salad
1 order
410 Calories
🍞

APPLEBEE'S
Teriyaki Shrimp Pasta
1 order
440 Calories

APPLEBEE'S
Teriyaki Chicken Pasta
1 order
450 Calories

ALL-AMERICAN DIET

Build-a-Meal
Applebee's

Low Carb= **Sodium Controlled=** **Vegetarian=**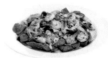

APPLEBEE'S
Grilled Dijon Chicken and
Portobello
1 order
470 Calories

APPLEBEE'S
Weight Watchers Chipotle
Lime Chicken
1 order
490 Calories

APPLEBEE'S
Grilled Shrimp and
Spinach Salad without
Dressing
1 order
680 Calories

Build-a-Meal
Blimpie

Low Carb= 🍞 **Sodium Controlled=** 🧂 **Vegetarian=** 🥕

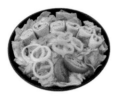

BLIMPIE
Buffalo Chicken Salad
1 order
220 Calories

🍞

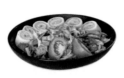

BLIMPIE
Ultimate Club Salad
1 order
260 Calories

🍞

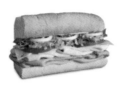

BLIMPIE
6″ Club
1 sandwich
410 Calories

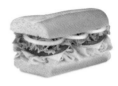

BLIMPIE
6″ Turkey and Provolone
1 sandwich
410 Calories

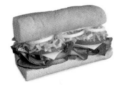

BLIMPIE
6″ Ham and Swiss
1 sandwich
420 Calories

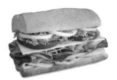

BLIMPIE
6″ Roast Beef and
Provolone
1 sandwich
430 Calories

BLIMPIE
6″ Blimpie Best
1 sandwich
450 Calories

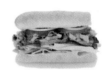

BLIMPIE
6″ Blimpie Trio
1 sandwich
510 Calories

BLIMPIE
Southwestern Wrap
1 wrap
530 Calories

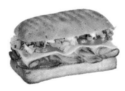

BLIMPIE
Buffalo Chicken on
Ciabatta
1 sandwich
540 Calories

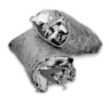

BLIMPIE
Chicken Caesar Wrap
1 wrap
560 Calories

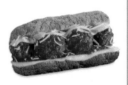

BLIMPIE
6″ Meatball
1 sandwich
580 Calories

ALL-AMERICAN DIET

Build-a-Meal
Blimpie

Low Carb= 🧂 **Sodium Controlled=** 📱 **Vegetarian=** 🌿

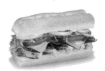

BLIMPIE
6″ Chicken Cheddar
Bacon Ranch
1 sandwich
600 Calories

DIET DETECTIVE WHAT YOU NEED TO KNOW

THE STRESS AND FAT CONNECTION

Deadlines, bills, gridlock, kids screaming—you face sources of stress every day. The physical problems arising from the effects of day-to-day stress range from mildly annoying (gray hair, wrinkles, occasional memory lapses) to debilitating (insomnia, poor eating habits, life-threatening diseases). And yes, it's true: Stress can cause you to gain weight. Here are a few tips to help you relax and stay healthy during stressful times.

1. **Create a "Stress Snack Eating" Kit.** Create a kit filled with portion-controlled low-calorie snacks to keep in your office or at home to break out when needed. Also, put in a few non-food items, such as an iPod loaded with comedy sketches and a jump-rope.

2. **Keep Unhealthy Snacks Out of Sight.** Researchers have shown time and again that snacks you can see are snacks that you eat.

3. **Come Up with Healthy Comfort Foods.** My favorite is popcorn.

4. **Develop a Stress-Eating Alternate Action Plan.** Try to find enjoyable, nonfood-related activities that can distract you: exercising, shopping, going to the movies, using relaxation techniques, working, chatting with friends, reading a humorous book. Have your plan in place before the stressful situation takes control.

5. **Exercise the Stress Away.** Go out for a walk, take a spin class, go for a run. Physical activity increases endorphins (the brain chemicals that control mood).

6. **Write Down Your Emotional Eating Triggers.** Write down your most common stress-causing situations. From this record, you can identify some of the triggers that may lead to overeating and then work to manage your behavior.

Build-a-Meal
Burger King

Low Carb= 🍞 **Sodium Controlled=** 🧂 **Vegetarian=** 🥕

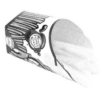

BURGER KING
Fresh Apple Fries with
Caramel Sauce
1 order
70 Calories
🧂 🥕

BURGER KING
Cheeseburger
1 sandwich
300 Calories

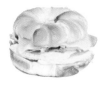

BURGER KING
Ham, Egg and Cheese
Croissan'wich
1 sandwich
350 Calories

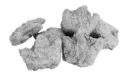

BURGER KING
8-Piece Chicken Tenders
1 order
380 Calories

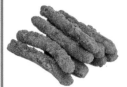

BURGER KING
9-Piece Chicken Fries
1 order
380 Calories

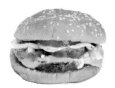

BURGER KING
Whopper Jr. with Cheese
1 sandwich
390 Calories

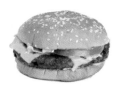

BURGER KING
Veggie Burger with
Cheese
1 sandwich
450 Calories
🥕

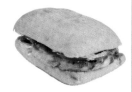

BURGER KING
Tendergrill Chicken Sand-
wich on Ciabatta
1 sandwich
470 Calories

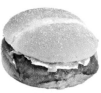
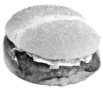

BURGER KING
Fish Sandwich
1 sandwich
640 Calories

Build-a-Meal
Chili's

Low Carb= **Sodium Controlled=** **Vegetarian=**

CHILI'S
Guacamole
1 order
45 Calories

CHILI'S
Side of Broccoli
1 order
80 Calories

CHILI'S
Spicy Garlic and Lime
Shrimp
6 pieces
150 Calories

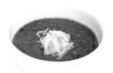

CHILI'S
Cup of Terlingua Chili
with Toppings
1 order
180 Calories

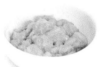

CHILI'S
Cinnamon Apples
1 order
280 Calories

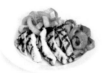

CHILI'S
Grilled Chicken Fajita
without Tortilla &
Condiments
1 order
360 Calories

CHILI'S
Classic Sirloin
1 order
360 Calories

CHILI'S
Guiltless Grill Classic
Sirloin
1 order
370 Calories

CHILI'S
Loaded Mashed Potatoes
1 order
390 Calories

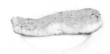

CHILI'S
Guiltless Grill Salmon with
Garlic and Herbs
1 order
480 Calories

CHILI'S
Margarita Grilled Chicken
1 order
550 Calories

CHILI'S
Guiltless Grill Grilled
Chicken Sandwich
1 sandwich
530 Calories

RESTAURANTS

Build-a-Meal
Chipotle Mexican Grill

Low Carb= 🍞 **Sodium Controlled=** 🧂 **Vegetarian=** 🥕

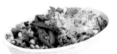

**CHIPOTLE
MEXICAN GRILL**
Veggie Burrito Bowl
1 order
400 Calories

**CHIPOTLE
MEXICAN GRILL**
Chopped Salad with
Black Beans, Chicken,
Salsa and Guacamole
1 order
490 Calories

DIET DETECTIVE WHAT YOU NEED TO KNOW

ACTION

Develop an action plan by thinking ahead. When pursuing a goal, it is crucial to have a well-thought-out, written plan. You can minimize crises by anticipating obstacles and planning for how you will surmount them. And keep in mind, great things are not achieved by impulse but by a series of small things—microchoices—that add up. Microchoices are the ones we make in the moment. For instance, whether we choose to eat an apple or a slice of apple pie, whether we bike to work or take the car. It's those microchoices that make up our lives. To learn more about microchoices see www.dietdetective.com/column/micro-choices.aspx. Also, confidence is critical for taking action: In fact, a study published in the *Journal of the American Dietetic Association* found that as self-efficacy improved, eating habits also improved and weight loss was greater. See www.dietdetective.com/column/confidence-to-lose.aspx.

Build-a-Meal
Denny's

Low Carb= 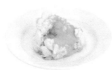 **Sodium Controlled=** **Vegetarian=**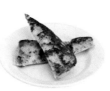

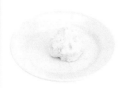

DENNY'S
Mashed Potatoes Plain
1 order
100 Calories

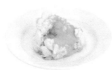

DENNY'S
Smoked Cheddar Mashed
Potatoes
1 side order
120 Calories

DENNY'S
Bacon
4 strips
140 Calories

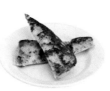

DENNY'S
Garlic Dinner Bread
2 pieces
170 Calories

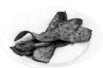

DENNY'S
Turkey Bacon
4 strips
180 Calories

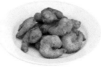

DENNY'S
Golden Fried Shrimp
6 pieces
190 Calories

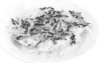

DENNY'S
Hash Browns
1 order
210 Calories

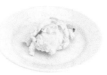

DENNY'S
Scrambled Eggs
2 eggs
250 Calories

DENNY'S
Hearty Wheat Pancakes
2 pancakes
310 Calories

DENNY'S
Grilled Chicken Salad
1 order
340 Calories

DENNY'S
Grilled Shrimp Skewers
4 skewers
360 Calories

DENNY'S
BLT Sandwich
1 sandwich
520 Calories

Build-a-Meal
Denny's

Low Carb= **Sodium Controlled=** **Vegetarian=**

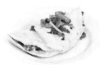

DENNY'S
Ultimate Omelette
1 omelette
620 Calories

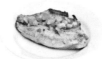

DENNY'S
Tilapia Ranchero with
Bread
1 order
630 Calories

DIET DETECTIVE WHAT YOU NEED TO KNOW

Create a responsible attitude right now; recognize that you are the only one who can make something happen in your life. People love to blame. We blame situations, circumstances, events, and even ourselves for where we are in our lives. Blame allows us to avoid taking a necessary action. It excuses us from acting responsibly. In terms of diet, it allows us to avoid focusing on controlling our weight because there's nothing we can do about it. Keep in mind, however, that one of the key characteristics of all successful weight losers is their ability to avoid blaming and accept responsibility for whatever failures or setbacks trip them up along the road. Keep this concept close to you when you attempt your next weight-loss campaign: We may not be fully responsible for every event in our lives; accidents do happen, both lucky and unlucky ones. However, we are solely responsible for how we respond to those events and how we allow them to shape us. Many of our own patterns—which we do control—bring us opportunity, success, and failure. See The Blame Game: How Your Behavior Might be Hindering Your Weight Control at www.dietdetective.com/columns/the-blame-game.aspx.

Build-a-Meal
Dunkin' Donuts

Low Carb= **Sodium Controlled=** **Vegetarian=**

DUNKIN' DONUTS
Shot of Espresso
1 shot
5 Calories

DUNKIN' DONUTS
Iced Black Coffee
1 16-ounce cup
10 Calories

DUNKIN' DONUTS
Black Coffee
1 14-ounce cup
10 Calories

DUNKIN' DONUTS
Iced Black Coffee
1 24-ounce cup
15 Calories

DUNKIN' DONUTS
Iced Coffee with Skim Milk
1 16-ounce cup
20 Calories

DUNKIN' DONUTS
Iced Coffee with Skim Milk
and Splenda
1 24-ounce cup
40 Calories

DUNKIN' DONUTS
Coffee with Cream
1 10-ounce cup
60 Calories

DUNKIN' DONUTS
Glazed Chocolate
Cake Munchkin
1 Munchkin
70 Calories

DUNKIN' DONUTS
Glazed Munchkin
1 munchkin
70 Calories

DUNKIN' DONUTS
Lite Latte
1 10-ounce cup
80 Calories

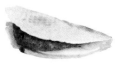

DUNKIN' DONUTS
Egg White Turkey Sau-
sage and Cheese
Wake Up Wrap
1 sandwich
150 Calories

DUNKIN' DONUTS
Lite Latte
1 24-ounce cup
160 Calories

RESTAURANTS

Build-a-Meal
Dunkin' Donuts

Low Carb= 🍞 **Sodium Controlled=** 🧂 **Vegetarian=** 🥕

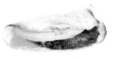

DUNKIN' DONUTS
Sausage, Egg and
Cheese Wrap
1 wrap
290 Calories

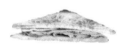

DUNKIN' DONUTS
Turkey, Cheddar and
Bacon Flatbread
Sandwich
1 sandwich
410 Calories

Build-a-Meal
Jamba Juice

Low Carb= **Sodium Controlled=** **Vegetarian=**

JAMBA JUICE
Steel Cut Oatmeal, Plain
1 order
220 Calories

JAMBA JUICE
Caribbean Passion
Smoothie
1 16-ounce cup
250 Calories

JAMBA JUICE
Strawberry Nirvana Light
Smoothie
1 30-ounce cup
300 Calories

JAMBA JUICE
Steel Cut Oatmeal, Apple
Cinnamon, No Brown
Sugar
1 order
360 Calories

JAMBA JUICE
Steel Cut Oatmeal,
Blackberry and Blueberry
with Brown Sugar
1 order
390 Calories

JAMBA JUICE
Banana Berry Smoothie
1 20-ounce cup
400 Calories

RESTAURANTS

Build-a-Meal
KFC

Low Carb= 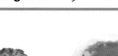 **Sodium Controlled=** **Vegetarian=**

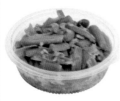

KFC
Green Beans
1 order
25 Calories

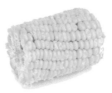

KFC
3″ Corn on the Cob
1 piece
70 Calories

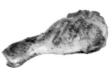

KFC
Grilled Drumstick
1 piece
90 Calories

KFC
Mashed Potatoes
and Gravy
1 order
120 Calories

KFC
5.5″ Corn on the Cob
1 piece
140 Calories

KFC
Coleslaw
1 order
150 Calories

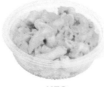

KFC
Macaroni and Cheese
1 order
160 Calories

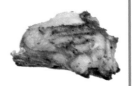

KFC
Grilled Thigh
1 piece
170 Calories

KFC
Biscuit
1 biscuit
180 Calories

KFC
Grilled Breast
1 piece
220 Calories

KFC
Potato Wedges
1 order
290 Calories

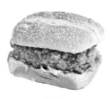

KFC
Extra Crispy Snacker
1 sandwich
310 Calories

Build-a-Meal
KFC

Low Carb=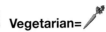 Sodium Controlled=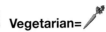 Vegetarian=

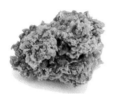

KFC
Extra Crispy Thigh
1 piece
340 Calories

KFC
Individual Popcorn
Chicken
1 order
400 Calories

KFC
Original Recipe Drumstick
Value Box
1 order
400 Calories

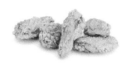

KFC
Hot Wings Value Box
1 order
490 Calories

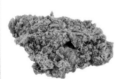

KFC
Extra Crispy Breast
1 piece
510 Calories

KFC
Original Recipe Thigh
Value Box
1 order
540 Calories

Build-a-Meal
McDonald's

Low Carb= **Sodium Controlled=** **Vegetarian=**

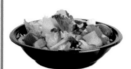

MCDONALD'S
Side Salad
1 order
20 Calories

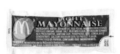

MCDONALD'S
Light Mayonnaise
1 packet
45 Calories

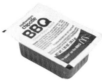

MCDONALD'S
Southwestern Chipotle
BBQ Sauce
1 container
50 Calories

MCDONALD'S
Butter Garlic Croutons
1 pouch
60 Calories

MCDONALD'S
Caramel Dip
1 container
70 Calories

MCDONALD'S
Newman's Own
Southwest Dressing
1 packet
100 Calories

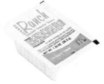

MCDONALD'S
Creamy Ranch Sauce
1 container
110 Calories

MCDONALD'S
Vanilla Ice Cream Cone
1 cone
150 Calories

MCDONALD'S
Fruit 'n Yogurt Parfait
1 parfait
160 Calories

MCDONALD'S
Newman's Own Ranch
Dressing
1 packet
170 Calories

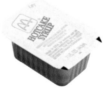

MCDONALD'S
Hotcake Syrup
1 container
180 Calories

MCDONALD'S
Newman's Own Creamy
Caesar Dressing
1 packet
190 Calories

Build-a-Meal
McDonald's

Low Carb= Sodium Controlled= Vegetarian=

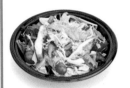

MCDONALD'S
Premium Caesar Salad
with Grilled Chicken
1 order
190 Calories

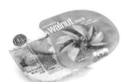

MCDONALD'S
Snack Size
Fruit & Walnut Salad
1 order
210 Calories

MCDONALD'S
Small Fries
1 order
230 Calories

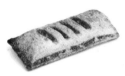

MCDONALD'S
Baked Apple Pie
1 piece
250 Calories

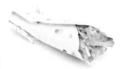

MCDONALD'S
Grilled Chicken Chipotle
BBQ Snack Wrap
1 wrap
250 Calories

MCDONALD'S
Strawberry Sundae
1 sundae
280 Calories

MCDONALD'S
Fruit and Maple Oatmeal
1 order
290 Calories

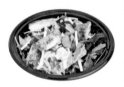

MCDONALD'S
Premium Southwest
Salad with Grilled Chicken
1 order
290 Calories

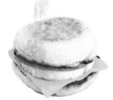

MCDONALD'S
Egg McMuffin
1 sandwich
300 Calories

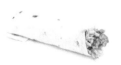

MCDONALD'S
Crispy Chicken Honey
Mustard Snack Wrap
1 wrap
330 Calories

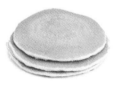

MCDONALD'S
Hotcakes
1 order
350 Calories

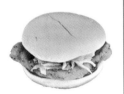

MCDONALD'S
McChicken Sandwich,
no mayo
1 sandwich
360 Calories

RESTAURANTS

Build-a-Meal
McDonald's

Low Carb= 🍞 **Sodium Controlled=** 🧂 **Vegetarian=** 🥕

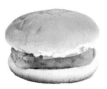

MCDONALD'S
Filet-O-Fish
with tartar sauce
1 sandwich
380 Calories

MCDONALD'S
Medium Fries
1 order
380 Calories

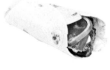

MCDONALD'S
Angus Deluxe
Snack Wrap
1 wrap
410 Calories

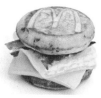

MCDONALD'S
Bacon Egg Cheese
McGriddle
1 sandwich
420 Calories

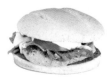

MCDONALD'S
Premium Grilled Chicken
Classic Sandwich
1 sandwich
420 Calories

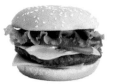

MCDONALD'S
Big 'N Tasty
1 sandwich
460 Calories

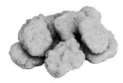

MCDONALD'S
10-Piece Chicken
McNuggets
1 order
470 Calories

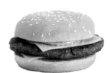

MCDONALD'S
Quarter Pounder
with Cheese
1 sandwich
510 Calories

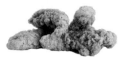

MCDONALD'S
5-Piece Chicken Selects
1 order
640 Calories

Build-a-Meal
Olive Garden

Low Carb= Sodium Controlled= Vegetarian=

OLIVE GARDEN
Marinara Sauce
1 order
35 Calories

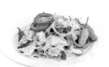

OLIVE GARDEN
Garden Salad,
No Dressing
1 order
120 Calories

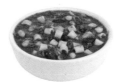

OLIVE GARDEN
Pasta e Fagioli Soup
1 bowl
130 Calories

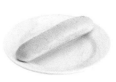

OLIVE GARDEN
Breadstick
1 breadstick
150 Calories

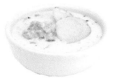

OLIVE GARDEN
Zuppa Toscana
1 bowl
170 Calories

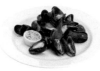

OLIVE GARDEN
Mussels di Napoli
1 order
180 Calories

OLIVE GARDEN
Italian Salad Dressing
1 container
230 Calories

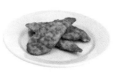

OLIVE GARDEN
Chicken Fingers Appetizer
3 pieces
330 Calories

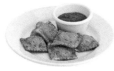

OLIVE GARDEN
Toasted Beef
& Pork Ravioli
6 pieces
360 Calories

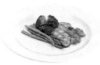

OLIVE GARDEN
Venetian Apricot Chicken
1 order
400 Calories

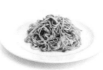

OLIVE GARDEN
Linguine alla Marinara
1 order
430 Calories

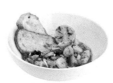

OLIVE GARDEN
Seafood Brodetto
1 order
480 Calories

Build-a-Meal
Olive Garden

Low Carb= 🍞 **Sodium Controlled=** 🧂 **Vegetarian=** 🌿

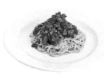

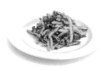

OLIVE GARDEN
Capellini Pomodoro
(specify lunch size)
1 order
480 Calories

OLIVE GARDEN
Penne Rigate
with Marinara
1 order
520 Calories

OLIVE GARDEN
Parmesan Crusted Tilapia
with Veggies
1 order
590 Calories

ALL-AMERICAN DIET

Build-a-Meal
P.F. Chang's

Low Carb= **Sodium Controlled=** **Vegetarian=**

P.F. CHANG'S
Fortune Cookie
1 cookie
30 Calories

P.F. CHANG'S
Steamed Vegetable
Dumplings
1 serving
45 Calories

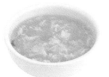

P.F. CHANG'S
Egg Drop Soup
1 cup
60 Calories

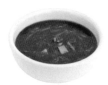

P.F. CHANG'S
Hot and Sour Soup
1 cup
80 Calories

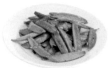

P.F. CHANG'S
Garlic Snap Peas
1 small order
96 Calories

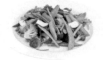

P.F. CHANG'S
Steamed Buddha's Feast
1 order
110 Calories

P.F. CHANG'S
Sichuan Style Asparagus
1 order
150 Calories

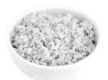

P.F. CHANG'S
Brown Rice
1 order
190 Calories

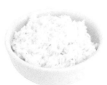

P.F. CHANG'S
White Rice
1 order
220 Calories

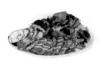

P.F. CHANG'S
Seared Ahi Tuna
1 order
320 Calories

P.F. CHANG'S
Shanghai Shrimp with
Garlic Sauce
1 order
390 Calories

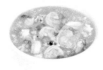

P.F. CHANG'S
Shrimp
with Lobster Sauce
1 order
500 Calories

Build-a-Meal
P.F. Chang's

Low Carb= 🍞 **Sodium Controlled=** 🧂 **Vegetarian=** 🌶

P.F. CHANG'S
Sichuan Shrimp
1 order
519 Calories

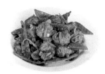

P.F. CHANG'S
Orange Peel Shrimp
1 order
561 Calories

ALL-AMERICAN DIET

Build-a-Meal
Pizza Hut

Low Carb= Sodium Controlled= Vegetarian=

PIZZA HUT
6-Piece All American
Traditional Chicken Wings
1 order
240 Calories

PIZZA HUT
Veggie Lover's Personal
Pan Pizza
1 pizza
550 Calories

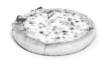

PIZZA HUT
Cheese Personal
Pan Pizza
1 pizza
590 Calories

Build-a-Meal
Quiznos

Low Carb= 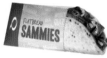 **Sodium Controlled=** 🧂 **Vegetarian=** 🥕

QUIZNOS
Chicken Noodle Soup
1 bowl
115 Calories

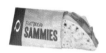

QUIZNOS
Q-Kidz Ham & Cheese
Bistro Sammie
1 sandwich
200 Calories

QUIZNOS
Chili
1 bowl
235 Calories

🧂

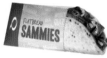

QUIZNOS
Roadhouse Steak
Sammie
1 sandwich
270 Calories

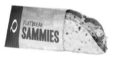

QUIZNOS
Cantina Chicken Bistro
Sammie
1 sandwich
280 Calories

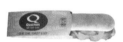

QUIZNOS
Q Kidz Ham & Cheese
1 sandwich
310 Calories

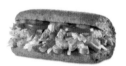

QUIZNOS
6˝ Honey Bourbon
Chicken
1 sandwich
320 Calories

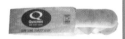

QUIZNOS
Q Kidz Cheesy Toasted
Cheese Bistro Sammie
1 sandwich
330 Calories

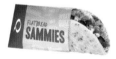

QUIZNOS
Veggie Sammie
1 sandwich
340 Calories

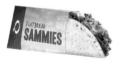

QUIZNOS
Italiano Flatbread Sammie
1 sandwich
370 Calories

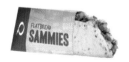

QUIZNOS
Chicken Bacon Ranch
Bistro Flatbread Sammie
1 sandwich
380 Calories

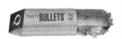

QUIZNOS
Pesto Turkey Bullet
1 sandwich
380 Calories

ALL-AMERICAN DIET

Build-a-Meal
Quiznos

Low Carb= 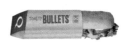 **Sodium Controlled=** **Vegetarian=**

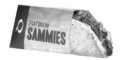

QUIZNOS
Bistro Steak Melt Sammie
1 sandwich
390 Calories

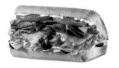

QUIZNOS
6″ The Traditional
1 sandwich
430 Calories

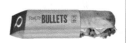

QUIZNOS
Beef, Bacon & Cheddar
Bullet
1 sandwich
450 Calories

QUIZNOS
Turkey Club Bullet
1 sandwich
460 Calories

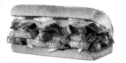

QUIZNOS
6″ Baja Chicken
1 sandwich
490 Calories

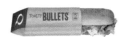

QUIZNOS
Italian Bullet
1 sandwich
500 Calories

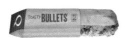

QUIZNOS
Tuna Melt Bullet
1 sandwich
510 Calories

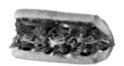

QUIZNOS
6″ Classic Italian
1 sandwich
520 Calories

RESTAURANTS

Build-a-Meal
Rally's/Checkers

Low Carb= **Sodium Controlled=** 🧂 **Vegetarian=** 🌶️

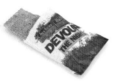

RALLY'S/CHECKERS
Cinnamon Apple Pie
1 piece
240 Calories
🌶️

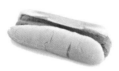

RALLY'S/CHECKERS
All Beef Hot Dog
1 hot dog
280 Calories

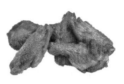

RALLY'S/CHECKERS
5-Piece Medium
Buffalo Wings
1 order
335 Calories

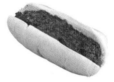

RALLY'S/CHECKERS
Medium Fries
1 order
350 Calories

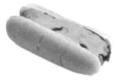

RALLY'S/CHECKERS
Chili Cheese Dog
1 hot dog
380 Calories

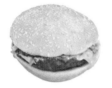

RALLY'S/CHECKERS
Checkerburger with
Cheese
1 sandwich
400 Calories

RALLY'S/CHECKERS
Large Fries
1 order
400 Calories

RALLY'S/CHECKERS
Chili Dog
1 hot dog
410 Calories

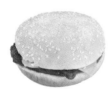

RALLY'S/CHECKERS
The All-American
Cheeseburger
1 sandwich
460 Calories

RALLY'S/CHECKERS
Double Checkerburger
with Cheese
1 sandwich
530 Calories

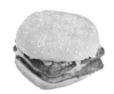

RALLY'S/CHECKERS
Deep Sea Double
1 sandwich
640 Calories

ALL-AMERICAN DIET

Build-a-Meal
Red Lobster

Low Carb= **Sodium Controlled=** **Vegetarian=**

RED LOBSTER
Live Maine Lobster
1 order
45 Calories

RED LOBSTER
Fresh Asparagus
1 order
60 Calories

RED LOBSTER
Garden Salad
without Dressing
1 order
90 Calories

RED LOBSTER
Chilled Jumbo Shrimp
Cocktail
1 order
120 Calories

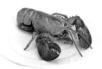

RED LOBSTER
Salmon with Fresh
Broccoli
1 order
270 Calories

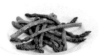

RED LOBSTER
Broiled Seafood Platter
1 order
300 Calories

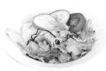

RED LOBSTER
Sailor's Platter
1 order
330 Calories

RED LOBSTER
Tilapia with Fresh Broccoli
1 order
360 Calories

RED LOBSTER
Garlic Grilled
Jumbo Shrimp
1 order
370 Calories

RED LOBSTER
Rainbow Trout
with Fresh Broccoli
1 order
410 Calories

RED LOBSTER
Wood-Grilled Lobster,
Shrimp and Scallops
1 order
500 Calories

Build-a-Meal
Ruby Tuesday

Low Carb= **Sodium Controlled=** **Vegetarian=**

RUBY TUESDAY
Fresh Grilled Green Beans
1 order
45 Calories

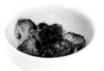

RUBY TUESDAY
Side of Broccoli
1 order
91 Calories

RUBY TUESDAY
Berry Good Yogurt Parfait
1 parfait
162 Calories

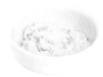

RUBY TUESDAY
Side of White Cheddar
Mashed Potatoes
1 order
223 Calories

RUBY TUESDAY
Chicken Tender Dinner
1 order
376 Calories

RUBY TUESDAY
Chicken Florentine
1 order
378 Calories

RUBY TUESDAY
Top Sirloin
1 order
392 Calories

RUBY TUESDAY
Asian Glazed Salmon
1 order
417 Calories

RUBY TUESDAY
Garden Salad with Light
Ranch Dressing
1 order
446 Calories

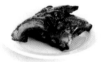

RUBY TUESDAY
Classic Barbecue
Half-Rack Ribs
1 order
500 Calories

RUBY TUESDAY
Trout Almondine
1 order
560 Calories

RUBY TUESDAY
Grilled Salmon
with mashed potatoes
and broccoli
1 order
664 Calories

ALL-AMERICAN DIET

Build-a-Meal
Starbucks

Low Carb= **Sodium Controlled=** **Vegetarian=**

STARBUCKS
Grande Black Coffee
1 16-ounce cup
5 Calories

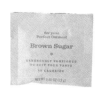

STARBUCKS
Brown Sugar for
Perfect Oatmeal
1 packet
50 Calories

STARBUCKS
Tall Iced Black Coffee,
Sweetened
1 12-ounce cup
60 Calories

STARBUCKS
Deluxe Fruit Blend
1 container
90 Calories

STARBUCKS
Tall Iced Coffee
with Whole Milk,
Sweetened
1 12-ounce cup
90 Calories

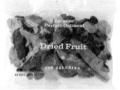

STARBUCKS
Dried Fruit Topping for
Perfect Oatmeal
1 pouch
100 Calories

STARBUCKS
Nut Medley Topping for
Perfect Oatmeal
1 pouch
100 Calories

STARBUCKS
Tall Nonfat Latte
1 12-ounce cup
100 Calories

STARBUCKS
Venti Nonfat Cappuccino
1 20-ounce cup
110 Calories

STARBUCKS
Tall Caramel Frappuccino
Light Blended Beverage
1 12-ounce cup
130 Calories

STARBUCKS
Perfect Oatmeal, Plain
1 order
140 Calories

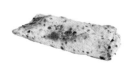

STARBUCKS
Spinach, Egg White
& Feta Wrap
1 wrap
280 Calories

Build-a-Meal
Starbucks

Low Carb= Sodium Controlled= Vegetarian=

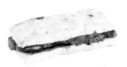

STARBUCKS
Roasted Vegetable Panini
1 panini
350 Calories

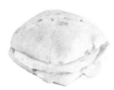

STARBUCKS
Veggie, Egg and
Monterey Jack Artisan
Breakfast Sandwich
1 sandwich
350 Calories

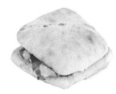

STARBUCKS
Bacon and Gouda Artisan
Breakfast Sandwich
1 sandwich
350 Calories

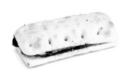

STARBUCKS
Roasted Tomato and
Mozzarella Sandwich
1 panini
380 Calories

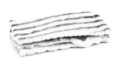

STARBUCKS
Chicken Santa Fe Panini
1 panini
400 Calories

STARBUCKS
Tarragon Chicken Salad
Sandwich
1 sandwich
420 Calories

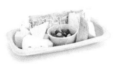

STARBUCKS
Cheese and Fruit Bistro
Box
1 container
460 Calories

Build-a-Meal
Subway

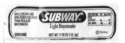

SUBWAY
Light Mayonnaise
1 packet
50 Calories

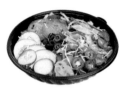

SUBWAY
Oven Roasted Chicken
Breast Salad
1 order
130 Calories

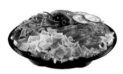

SUBWAY
Baked Lay's
1 bag
130 Calories

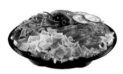

SUBWAY
Club Salad
1 order
140 Calories

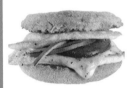

SUBWAY
Egg White and Cheese
on Light Wheat English
Muffin
1 sandwich
150 Calories

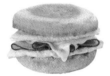

SUBWAY
Egg White & Cheese with
Ham on Light Wheat
English Muffin
1 sandwich
160 Calories

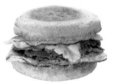

SUBWAY
Steak, Egg and Cheese
on Light WheatEnglish
Muffin
1 sandwich
200 Calories

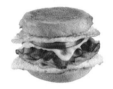

SUBWAY
Sunrise Melt with Egg
Whites on Light Wheat-
English Muffin
1 sandwich
210 Calories

SUBWAY
Sun Chips Harvest
Cheddar
1 bag
210 Calories

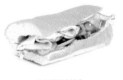

SUBWAY
6″ Veggie Delight
on Italian
1 sandwich
220 Calories

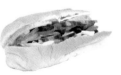

SUBWAY
6″ Veggie Delight
Sandwich on White
1 sandwich
230 Calories

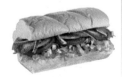

SUBWAY
6″ Turkey Breast
Sandwich on White
1 sandwich
270 Calories

RESTAURANTS

Build-a-Meal
Subway

Low Carb= **Sodium Controlled=** **Vegetarian=**

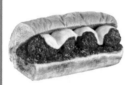

SUBWAY
Roasted Chicken
Noodle Soup
1 bowl
310 Calories

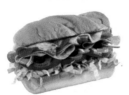

SUBWAY
6″ Spicy Italian on Italian
1 sandwich
510 Calories

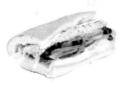

SUBWAY
6″ Tuna Sandwich
on Italian
1 sandwich
520 Calories

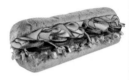

SUBWAY
Footlong Turkey Breast on
9-Grain Wheat
1 sandwich
550 Calories

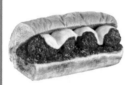

SUBWAY
6″ Meatball Marinara on
Italian
1 sandwich
570 Calories

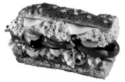

SUBWAY
6″ Tuna on Honey Oat
1 sandwich
580 Calories

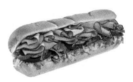

SUBWAY
Footlong Black Forest
Ham on Italian
1 sandwich
590 Calories

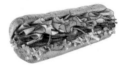

SUBWAY
Footlong Turkey and Ham
on Wheat
1 sandwich
610 Calories

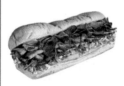

SUBWAY
Footlong Roast Beef
on Italian
1 sandwich
650 Calories

ALL-AMERICAN DIET

Build-a-Meal
Taco Bell

Low Carb= Sodium Controlled= Vegetarian=

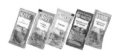

TACO BELL
Variety Hot Sauces
1 packet
0 Calories

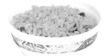

TACO BELL
Mexican Rice
1 order
120 Calories

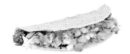

TACO BELL
Fresco Beef Crunchy Taco
1 taco
150 Calories

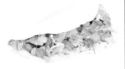

TACO BELL
Fresco Chicken Soft Taco
1 taco
150 Calories

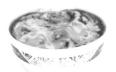

TACO BELL
Pintos and Cheese
1 order
170 Calories

TACO BELL
Cheese Roll-Up
1 order
190 Calories

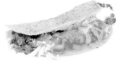

TACO BELL
Crunchy Taco Supreme
1 taco
200 Calories

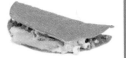

TACO BELL
Volcano Taco
1 taco
230 Calories

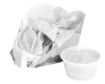

TACO BELL
Cheesy Nachos
1 order
280 Calories

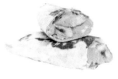

TACO BELL
Grilled Chicken Taquito
1 taquito
320 Calories

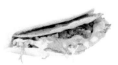

TACO BELL
Double Decker Taco
1 taco
320 Calories

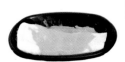

TACO BELL
Beef Enchirito
1 Enchirito
360 Calories

Build-a-Meal
Taco Bell

Low Carb= 🍞 **Sodium Controlled=** 🧂 **Vegetarian=** 🥕

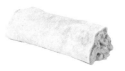

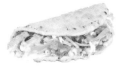

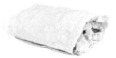

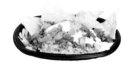

TACO BELL
Bean Burrito
1 burrito
370 Calories
🥕

TACO BELL
Baja Chicken Chalupa
1 chalupa
390 Calories
🍞

TACO BELL
Grilled Chicken Burrito
1 burrito
430 Calories

TACO BELL
Nachos Supreme
1 order
440 Calories
🍞

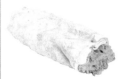

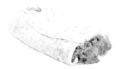

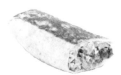

TACO BELL
½ Pound Combo Burrito
1 burrito
460 Calories

TACO BELL
7-Layer Burrito
1 burrito
500 Calories

TACO BELL
XXL Grilled Stuft Burrito—
Steak
1 burrito
820 Calories

Build-a-Meal
Wendy's

Low Carb= 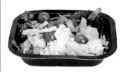 **Sodium Controlled=** **Vegetarian=**

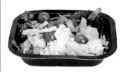

WENDY'S
Side Garden Salad,
no dressing
1 order
25 Calories

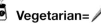

WENDY'S
Barbecue Sauce
1 container
45 Calories

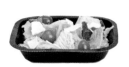

WENDY'S
Caesar Side Salad,
no dressing
1 order
60 Calories

WENDY'S
Marzetti Pomegranate
Vinaigrette Dressing
1 packet
60 Calories

WENDY'S
Marzetti Fat-Free French
Style Dressing
1 packet
40 Calories

WENDY'S
Gourmet Croutons
1 pouch
80 Calories

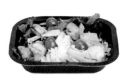

WENDY'S
Garden Side Salad with
Croutons
1 order
105 Calories

WENDY'S
Marzetti Lemon Garlic
Caesar Dressing
1 packet
110 Calories

WENDY'S
Small Chili
1 order
210 Calories

WENDY'S
5-Piece Chicken Nuggets
1 order
220 Calories

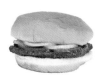

WENDY'S
Jr. Hamburger
1 sandwich
230 Calories

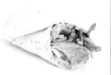

WENDY'S
Grilled Chicken Go Wrap
1 wrap
260 Calories

Build-a-Meal
Wendy's

Low Carb= **Sodium Controlled=** 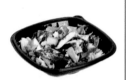 **Vegetarian=**

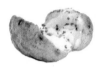

WENDY'S
Baked Potato, no topping
1 order
270 Calories

WENDY'S
Jr. Cheeseburger
1 sandwich
270 Calories

WENDY'S
Small French Fries
1 order
320 Calories

WENDY'S
Apple Pecan
Chicken Salad
1 order
340 Calories

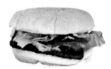

WENDY'S
Jr. Bacon Cheeseburger
1 sandwich
350 Calories

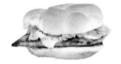

WENDY'S
Ultimate Chicken
Grill Sandwich
1 sandwich
360 Calories

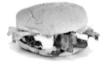

WENDY'S
Double Jr. Bacon
Cheeseburger
1 sandwich
440 Calories

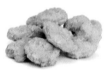

WENDY'S
10-Piece Chicken
Nuggets
1 order
450 Calories

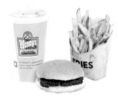

WENDY'S
Hamburger Kids' Meal
with Diet Soda
1 meal
450 Calories

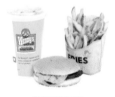

WENDY'S
Cheeseburger Kids' Meal
with Diet Soda
1 meal
490 Calories

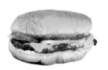

WENDY'S
¼ lb Single
Cheeseburger
1 sandwich
550 Calories

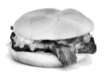

WENDY'S
Single Baconator
1 sandwich
620 Calories

ALL-AMERICAN DIET

230

Maintain Your Weight Loss

You've Lost the Weight! What Now?

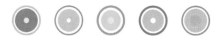

Congratulations! You made it. Now it's time to move on to *The Diet Detective's All-American Diet* maintenance program. It's pretty simple. The first thing you're going to do is figure out your new calorie needs based on your current weight and activity level. This time I would like you to use a more detailed formula than the one you used when you started. It will be based on a combination of your resting metabolic rate (RMR)—the number of calories you burn just to remain alive and keep your body functioning—and your activity level.

To determine how many calories you're burning through activity, you will choose from a predetermined scale ranging from "sedentary" to "extreme activity." Sedentary activities include sitting, driving, lying down, or standing in one place for most of the day and not doing any type of exercise. If you are sedentary, you still burn about 20 percent more calories than the calorie requirement based solely on your RMR. Extreme activities include heavy manual labor, army or Marine recruit training, or competitive athletics. If you are this active, you can eat more than double the calories required simply to maintain your body weight when you're at rest.

The following is the most widely accepted method of determining your calorie needs (*Source:* Harris-Benedict Equation):

Step 1: Calculate your resting metabolic rate (RMR).

Female: 655.1 + (4.35 × weight in pounds) + (4.699 × height in inches)– (4.676 × age)

Male: 66.5 + (6.25 × weight in pounds) + (12.71 × height in inches)–(6.775 × age)

Step 2: Calculate your calorie needs

Now that you've determined your RMR, multiply that number by your activity factor:

- Sedentary: 1.2 (You sit, drive, lie down, or stand in one place for most of the day and don't do any type of exercise.)
- Light activity: 1.3 to 1.4 (You're sedentary for most of the day and do light activity, such as walking, for no more than 2 hours daily.)
- Moderate activity: 1.5 (You're on your feet most of the workday, with light lifting only, and do no structured exercise.)
- Very active: 1.6 to 1.7 (Your typical workday includes several hours of physical labor, such as light industry and construction-type jobs.)
- Extreme activity: 2 to 2.4 (You do heavy manual labor or army or Marine recruit training or are a competitive athlete.)

Your RMR multiplied by your activity factor is your total daily calorie allowance for weight maintenance. So do this:

RMR _____ × Activity Level _____ = _____ Calories Per Day to Maintain

You can find an online calculator that will do this math for you here: http://goo.gl/cKKMg.

You now have the number of calories you need to stick with in order to maintain your current weight. Remember, this calculation is based on the average person; it is possible that your own calorie needs are either higher or lower. Use the number you have as your starting point, but if you notice that you're either losing or gaining weight, adjust the total by 100 calories more or less (depending on whether you're losing or gaining). Continue to monitor your weight on a weekly basis until you achieve a calorie level that allows you to maintain a healthy weight.

Cook One Meal

This is also a good time to start working some more fresh foods into your diet by trying to cook at least one meal per day, preferably dinner.

You could probably keep on eating frozen and ready-to-eat foods for the rest of your life; however, many of these are high in sodium or other preservatives, and it's also good to incorporate more balance and options into your meal plan.

You can find easy-to-prepare, healthy, and tasty recipes online at Web sites such as Eatingwell.com and Cookinglight.com. Start with dishes you like that are also quick and easy. Most of the recipes on these Web sites include shopping lists and use ingredients that are easy to find.

When you're planning your homemade meals, be sure they fit into your new calorie levels. Here are a few other tips.

DIET DETECTIVE'S WHAT YOU NEED TO KNOW

BATCH COOK AND FREEZE

One of the most effective ways to ensure that you always have a healthy meal on hand at home is to pick 1 day a week and cook several meals at once. For instance, cook pork chops or chicken in large batches, freeze on cookie sheets, and then store in the freezer in a sealed container with waxed paper between the pieces. Or cook large batches of soup or stew and freeze them in individual portion sizes. Take out only as much as you need to reheat in the oven or microwave.

As an alternative to cooking entire meals ahead, just double or triple up on some basic building blocks that will speed you through future meals. Browning batches of ground beef and onions, poaching or grilling chicken, and baking potatoes ahead of time are easy ways to cut down on meal prep time. Even having a supply of chopped onion, carrots, or other precut vegetables in the freezer will make the cooking process a lot faster.

Monitor Your Weight

Remember to weigh yourself regularly. If you ever find yourself slipping (that is, starting to gain weight), simply cut 500 calories per day and you will be back on track! The popular misconception is that no more than 2 percent of dieters can actually maintain their weight loss over time. But that is actually a myth based on only one or two studies that are now decades old. The fact is that about 20 percent of people in the general population are successful at long-term weight-loss maintenance. Here are a few strategies you can use to make sure you're among that 20 percent.

Beware of the "Fast-Metabolism-I-Can-Eat-Whatever-I-Want" Club

Does this sound familiar? After losing those pounds, you suddenly feel that, magically, your body has changed, making you a charter member of the exclusive "fast-metabolism-I-can-eat-whatever-I-want" club. For the first few weeks in your new, fit body, you are confident that the weight is off for good. You indulge, and the diet you were on is now ancient history, because all along you knew you could never live on that diet for the rest of your life. Weight control is a forever process, so you need to create practices you can live with—forever.

Keep Your Pants On

The National Weight Loss Registry has determined that almost all successful weight-loss maintainers have some kind of "5-pound warning system"—a way of measuring and/or monitoring their weight before it gets out of control. It could be something as simple as keeping a "thin" pair of pants or a dress to try on periodically instead of getting on the scale, but they all have some way of knowing if they are slipping, and a backup plan to put into action as soon as they receive their warning.

Keep Walking

Walking is an important key not only to weight loss but also to long-term weight maintenance. The theory is that as you lose weight, you need something to compensate for the lower metabolism—that's right, you burn fewer calories as you lose weight. Walking and other physical activities keep your calorie-burning capacity high.

Make It Automatic

Successful maintainers have figured out ways to make their behaviors and choices second nature. It's based on the concept of automaticity—the subconscious ways we perform daily behaviors like brushing our teeth. The idea is to apply the same principle to your diet. Arrange your personal environment to maximize your chances of losing and maintaining your weight loss and minimize your chances of slipping up.

Keep It Consistent

According to research at Brown University Medical School, a major predictor of successful weight maintenance is dietary consistency. This means that those who maintain the same diet regimen across the week and year are more likely to maintain their weight loss over the following year than those who diet more strictly on weekdays and/or during nonholiday periods.

It's Easier Over Time

Automated behavior is essential for permanent weight control, but the good news is that, according to a study conducted by the National Weight Control Registry and reported in *Obesity Research,* once you've lost weight and maintained the lower weight for more than a few years, weight maintenance gets easier.

Remember to Eat Breakfast

The research shows that all successful dieters eat breakfast each morning, which most likely prevents them from overeating during the rest of the day.

Frequently
Asked Questions

Q: What if I'm at a fast-food outlet or a restaurant and there are only a few items from the book on the menu?

Don't panic. If you are at a restaurant and don't see your food choice listed on these pages, it's because we tried to choose foods that are healthier than others and tried to stick to those that we felt comfortable recommending. For instance, if there was a 350-calorie meal that was very high in saturated fat, it might not have made it on the menu. However, that's not to say that you can't have it if it fits into your calorie level for your meal plan. One note: Make sure that you plan your meal before you go to any fast-food or chain restaurant—all the nutritional information is on the company Web site. Don't ever wing it—plan in advance.

Q: What if the food that I want for lunch is listed under the dinner options?

That's fine as long as it's at the same calorie level.

Q: Can I have two 50-calorie snacks instead of a 100-calorie snack?

That's fine, too.

Q: Why does the book have a different calorie count than the product Web site?

Product nutritional information changes—the companies change product size, ingredients, and packaging. All these affect nutritional information. Also, there are instances in which the product Web site has one set of nutritional information and the product packaging has another. The good news is that most of the time it doesn't vary by too much—2 to 5 percent at the most. With this in mind, you should still be label conscious, keeping in mind serving size and servings per package when you buy. With *The Diet Detective's All-American Diet,* we made sure that nearly all the items we picked are full packages, meaning you can eat the entire container's contents. The reason? I wanted to make sure you're not tempted to eat more than the recommended portion. That is another reason why certain "favorite foods" are missing from the book. If the entire package serving size is higher than the assigned calorie level, then it did not make the cut.

Q: Is there any place that you can go online that has grocery nutritional information?

Freshdirect.com is a supermarket delivery service in New York City, but you can take advantage of its fabulous Web site no matter where you live. The site offers an impressive amount of nutritional information, arranged in whatever order you choose, for almost every single food in the supermarket. Look for details of every ingredient as well as the Nutrition Facts panel at no charge. Just be sure to input a valid New York City ZIP code when prompted (try 10011): www.freshdirect.com. Also, be sure to check the USDA database at www.nal.usda.gov/fnic/foodcomp/search/.

Q: What if I eat out frequently?

Try to be extra cautious, because eating out can be dangerous to your waistline, especially during the 21-Day Jump Start Program and the first 120 days of the diet. That said, here are a few tips to keep in mind if you don't have access to the calories of the foods and you want to make sure you're sticking to the plan.

- Say no to butter, mayo, tartar sauce, creamy dressings, and extra cheese.
- Use mustard, ketchup, salt, pepper, or vinegar as fat-free ways to season your food.
- In salads, watch the nuts, croutons, and other add-ons.
- Dressing for the salad should always be ordered on the side and sprinkled on with a fork.
- Chicken and fish can be good choices—but *only* if they are grilled or broiled, *not* breaded or deep-fried.
- Instead of cheese, opt for lettuce, tomato, and onion. Removing just one slice of cheese can save you about 100 calories.
- Order a salad or a broth-based soup to enjoy before your main meal (avoid

creamy soups and dressings). Either one will help to fill you up for very few calories so that you eat less of the fattening stuff.

- Get Chinese food steamed with the sauce on the side; try mixed vegetables or chicken and broccoli. Avoid egg rolls, fried rice, and deep-fried dishes like sweet and sour chicken, sesame chicken, or General Tso's chicken (more than 1,000 calories). And skip the duck sauce—just 2 tablespoons has 80 calories.
- Even nonfat frozen yogurt can be a no-no when you add toppings.
- Top your pizza with vegetables instead of meat, and ask for half the cheese. Skip the stuffed pizza and the baked ziti or lasagna.
- Potatoes sound healthy, but the calories in the toppings can add up—skip the butter, bacon, and sour cream. Try vegetables and a light sprinkle of cheese.
- Look for the "light" or "healthy" menu items.
- Ask how your dish is prepared, and don't be shy about requesting it prepared without oil or butter.
- Look for baked, grilled, or broiled choices, and stay away from fried foods.

Go to the Internet. Almost every restaurant has its menu available online; check it out before you go and make sure you come up with several low-calorie options. You should also call the restaurant and ask what dishes they recommend and whether the chef would prepare certain dishes in a more healthful way (with no oil or butter, no cream sauces, etc.)

Q: *What happens if I don't follow the meal plans exactly?*
There is a "fudge factor" of 10 to 20 calories per day—but that goes both ways. If you go over your calorie limit by 20 calories today, try to go under your limit by 20 calories tomorrow. Also, if you do eat too much, ever hear that expression "Don't sweat it"? Well, you should "sweat it off," actually.

Q: *I just pigged out at a holiday dinner. Do I have to start again?*
Congratulations—you're human. We all make mistakes, and pigging out while on a diet is not a failure. It's just a slipup, a temporary setback that you can overcome. All is not lost.

Overdoing it for one meal or even for a full day or two will not undo all your hard work. The first thing you need to do is get yourself back in gear. Come up with a Relapse Prevention Plan: Keep in mind that a slip doesn't have to become a fall, nor does a lapse have to become a relapse. Unsuccessful weight-maintainers tend to have an all-or-nothing attitude and view a single "bad" eating situation as verification that they just can't lose weight. Think in advance about situations and obstacles that might cause brief breakdowns, such as eating a bag of potato chips or a box of cookies, and have a plan. For instance, if you normally have difficulty staying on your diet when you go out to dinner or when you're visiting relatives, come up with strategies to avoid the slipup, as well as a plan of action to follow if you actually do slip up. Follow the tips below:

- Plan the rest of your day accordingly. Do *not* skip meals, but have a lighter dinner (and lunch, too, if you haven't eaten lunch yet). A bowl of cereal and skim milk works well for a light meal (measure your portion so you're not having hundreds of extra calories), as does a container of low- or nonfat yogurt with fruit, a big salad, a baked potato with broccoli, or even a sandwich on whole grain bread.
- Fit in an extra 20 to 30 minutes of exercise today and tomorrow. This will give you a head start as you're getting back on track.
- Think about what may have gone wrong. Did you let yourself get too hungry? Were you eating to fill an emotional need? Was the food sitting right in front of you, tempting you even though you weren't hungry? The more you learn about your behaviors and *why* you slip up, the better you can prevent those lapses.

Also, keep in mind that if you have frequent "pig-outs," there is probably something about your diet plan that you need to adjust. Evaluate, and ask yourself if your diet is too restrictive. If so, make the necessary adjustments.

Q: I'm having a very stressful week. What can I do?

It's been one of those weeks, hasn't it? Everyone's been getting on your nerves, you have a hundred things you need to take care of, and it just doesn't seem like there are enough hours in the day—I can relate. It's okay to have a bit of stress, but too much can create problems. In fact, a Finnish study reported in *Psychosomatic Medicine* found a direct association between work stress and excess weight. You might want to try a few relaxation techniques—maybe even take a "staycation."

Take a deep breath. Deep breathing is a great way to relax and calm down in order to relieve stress. Try this:

Step 1: Become aware of your breathing. Sit or lie down in a quiet room with one hand placed on your abdomen.

Step 2: As you inhale, your belly should expand slightly on its own. Try to relax your abdominal muscles—you'll get the most effective breathing from a relaxed abdomen. If possible, inhale and exhale through your nose only.

Step 3: The hand resting on your abdomen should rise with your belly as you inhale and fall as you exhale.

Make notes. Get out your notepad and get organized. Prioritize. Make a list of what you need to do. Writing everything down will allow you to be more efficient with your time and resources. Plus, you'll feel great when you can cross something off the list after it's done.

When you're feeling stressed or anxious, instead of eating, call a friend and vent. Listen to some relaxing music. Get some physical activity. Exercise causes your body to release endorphins, which can give you the feeling of a "natural high." Laugh more by renting a few funny movies or even a TV series you've never seen. Get more sleep—research shows that sleep keeps weight off and reduces disease.

Q: I can't control myself when I start eating—help!

Many people struggle with this. First of all, don't be a Diet Hero—keep unhealthy foods out of the house. Don't tempt yourself. Focus on eating more slowly so that you become more aware of your body's hunger and satiety. Allow at least 20 minutes for your brain to receive the message that your stomach is full. Also, eating slowly allows you to appreciate your food more.

- Eat large quantities of steamed green veggies with salt, pepper, and fresh garlic. Nothing like a nice dose of low-calorie, high-nutrient vegetables.
- Drink a big glass of water or have a cup of green tea. Drinking fluids can help fill you up. Also, many times we mistake thirst for hunger. This will help you determine whether you're really hungry.

- Brush your teeth. I know this might sound ridiculous to some, but it can work as a reminder that eating is over and give you a sense of completion. Also, you might not want to give up that fresh-brushed feeling by eating junk food.
- Throw the food away. Sometimes just tossing the food helps. I realize that this can be a waste of food, but drastic times sometimes call for drastic measures.

Control your portions.

Use a smaller plate. As simple as this sounds, it works. Studies have shown that people eat more when there's more on their plates, regardless of how hungry they feel. So put less on your plate, but trick your eyes into thinking you're eating more by using a smaller plate so that it looks full.

Never eat directly out of the container. It's hard to keep track of how much you are eating when you're just reaching in and stuffing the food into your mouth. Before you know it, the bag is empty. Instead, use a measuring cup and/or scale, and measure your cereal into a bowl, your rice onto your plate, your tuna salad, your potato chips, your strawberries . . . everything. Put away the rest, and only then sit down to eat.

Q: I have no motivation today to diet or exercise—do you have any secret weapons for me to use?

Yes, here are a few things you need to learn and use as part of your dieting strategy: life preservers, mental rehearsal, and finding the "why."

Life Preservers

Create Life Preservers that will help you lose weight for good. Researchers at Utrecht University in the Netherlands reported that those who believed they could control their eating and didn't blame being overweight on "bad genes" lost the most weight. It's called visualization—an imagined, meaningful, detailed vision of your life after you've reached your goal weight; a specific moment in time. It was a hot topic during the last Olympics—an athlete having a vision of crossing the finish line and winning the race before starting the event. I call these visions life preservers. Think of every emotional and physical detail of these future moments and reflect on them when you need help to get through the tough times or when you feel that you're losing sight of your goal. For example, if weight loss is your goal, imagine a thinner, healthier you running into your ex at the mall. Write up three life preservers, keep them handy, and read them often—they should be about 700 words each.

Mental Rehearsal

Almost all world-class athletes practice mental rehearsal. Haven't you ever heard the expression "Practice makes perfect"? The concept is to rehearse an upcoming event, but not on the field—in your mind. By doing this, you trick your brain into having an experience you didn't actually have. You need to rehearse your eating behaviors and choices before they take place—before you eat at your favorite restaurant, before you go to the office knowing that it's "doughnut Friday."

Here is a step-by-step guide to mental rehearsal.

> **Step 1:** Identify the occasion. Choose an eating situation you find difficult, whether it's traveling, unconscious eating, special occasions (weddings, family dinners), dining out, a midnight snack attack, etc. Develop a rough sketch of how you'd like to change your behavior in that scenario—include the thoughts, emotions, and actions you want in your "ideal" version.

> **Step 2:** Brainstorm. Shane Murphy, PhD, a professor of psychology at Western Connecticut State University and a former sports psychologist to the US Olympic team, recommends brainstorming all the negative events that could occur within that situation. For instance, if you have difficulty sticking to your diet when you're going out to dinner at your favorite restaurant, come up with all the possible complications you may encounter: the great bread, the stupendous blue cheese dressing, the fabulous crème brûlée, or even those pressuring comments from "food pushers." And don't forget to think about all the positive outcomes in which you make choices you are content with—that's the key, reminds Dr. Murphy.

> **Step 3:** Add detail. Be specific. Don't spare a thought, no matter how insignificant it might seem. Think how you would act and behave in your ideal scenario—you can even write it down to make it more concrete.

Step 4: Create the script. Now you're ready to come up with a step-by-step description of exactly what your ideal experience would actually be like. Be creative and thoughtful about the process. You must really understand the experience from beginning to end. Consciously visualize what it will take for you to get through this situation, and make sure to think about how you would react to all the possible negative scenarios, creating a positive outcome for each.

Step 5: Give it life. Once you have the general script down, go back to make the experience really come alive. "Keep in mind you want to use all your senses—see, feel, hear, and smell it," says Dr. Murphy. Make it as lifelike as possible—imagine it in 3-D. If you're a swimmer, smell the chlorine in the pool. For weight control, apply the same principles, including imagining the smells of the restaurant, whom you'll be with, who your server will be, and what everyone is going to say.

There are two types of mental practicing: external, in which you watch yourself in a movie, and internal, in which you see the event through your own eyes. Some experts recommend the internal approach for greater success, but either will be effective, so use whichever you prefer.

Step 6: Make it automatic. Rehearse your imagery often, including the night before the event and even just before it begins, to keep it fresh. What you're doing through mental rehearsal is creating new "automatic" responses to replace your previous patterns—the ones that have been holding you back from your weight loss. Just think about it. If you've always ordered dessert at a restaurant, you do it unconsciously because it's a habit. If you do nothing to change that pattern, you will continue to do the same thing. But if you rehearse a different outcome—for instance, ordering fruit, coffee, or no dessert at all—you will have created a new "automatic" response to the dessert menu.

Step 7: Rerun that scenario in your head whenever you find yourself about to live out the situation you've rehearsed. The details should be as familiar to you as the words and notes to your favorite song.

Step 8: After the event, no matter what the outcome, revise your imagery and try to repair any mistakes or setbacks.

Finding the "Why"

Why in the world do you want to lose weight? You'd better have a very clear and precise reason that will stand up to your most powerful excuses. It helps to find a good reason why. Don't just say "for my health," "to look better," "to feel better." Be specific—"I want to lose weight because I would like to be there for my grandchild's graduation in 30 years." Keep in mind, if you're not sure or you treat this glibly, there's a high likelihood that you will not achieve your weight-loss goal. Think you already know? Make sure. Then write it down. Here are a few other tips to help you find your "why."

Rough roads. If you haven't clearly defined your reason for wanting to lose weight, as soon as you run into complications or the going gets tough, it will be hard to convince yourself that it's worth continuing.

After all, why would you pick a baked apple over a piece of chocolate cake at your favorite restaurant? The idea is that if you think your motivation is to lower your cholesterol, and that's not compelling enough to stand up to the chocolate cake—well, the chocolate cake will win every time. But if, instead, you're choosing between chocolate cake and feeling good about yourself in shorts during your upcoming family vacation—and that is truly important—then maybe that baked apple might start looking good after all.

Be autonomous. How often have you done something because someone else wanted you to do it, especially when it comes to losing weight? We hear it from our doctors, friends, parents, and spouses who "mean well"—but then we go on a diet for the wrong reasons. "People mouth goals that someone else has set for them—and this is not a very stable basis for personal change." When someone else sets expectations for us, we are often compelled to rebel. How many times have you looked at a doughnut and said, "I don't care what my husband (or wife) thinks—I'm eating that Krispy Kreme."

In fact, research demonstrates a greater likelihood of success on any weight-loss program, including increased weight loss and weight maintenance, if the participant's motivation is autonomous. In other words, you need to want to do this for YOUR OWN reasons, not because someone else thinks you should or because you think it's "the right thing to do."

Is it really you? Make sure your reason for losing weight is personally important. Make sure that you care about it, and remember that your choices directly affect your reward. Don't rely on feelings of obligation or pressure to motivate you. If you end up saying things like "Oh, I shouldn't eat that—it's a 'bad' food," you're really not connected to your reward. "Your reward needs to be strong and internally integrated for it to be motivating."

Make it real. In order to find your reason why, you may need to think about what it will be like to actually lose weight. How will you feel? What will you look like? If you've never been at your goal weight, it might be hard to get in touch with the feelings and benefits of being that weight. Spend time considering your end result. Use self-reflection and visualization techniques and fantasize about realistic, but exciting, reasons for being in shape.

Come clean. Being honest with yourself is critical. Ask yourself probing questions. Get your mind thinking about what makes this goal important. Self-honesty is no simple task. It involves reflecting and then endorsing, not just accepting. Just saying words like "I want to be healthier" or "I want to look better" might not be enough. Those words are too broad. You need to ask yourself why you want to look better or be healthier—what does that mean to you? Does looking better mean you're more attractive to others? That you get compliments? Don't just say the benefits—explore them and break them down. Get to the roots. If looking better is your reward, break it down into what that actually means to you. For example, "By looking better, I will get compliments from others. This will increase my motivation and will increase my confidence, and this will make me feel better about who I am."

Don't worry about others. Often we feel guilty about our reward because it's not "politically or socially correct," says Heather Patrick, PhD, a nutrition professor at Baylor College of Medicine in Houston. Our goals are *our* goals. Whether they're about fitting into a great pair of pants or being able to strut around in a bathing suit, that's our own business. The only caveat is that your goals shouldn't be physically or mentally destructive to your or others. Patrick also cautions, "Be careful what you choose, because certain rewards are fleeting and will not last over the long haul. For instance, if your reward is to get more compliments by looking better, what happens when the compliments end?" She recommends picking rewards that will continually motivate you. They tend to be the most powerful. One example could be the ability to spend more active time with your family.

Write it down. "Create an advantage/disadvantage analysis—basically a list of all the advantages and disadvantages of losing weight and all of the advantages and disadvantages of *not* losing the weight. Create four columns," suggests Jim Afremow, PhD, a sports psychologist at Athletes' Performance in Tempe, Arizona. This allows you to define your "why" and clarify your thinking. "It helps when you see these in black and white, and the list will serve as a reminder." After you write up your list of rewards, look it over to see which ones are the most important, which ones are "autonomous," and which ones will keep you going when things get rough. Then, review your list throughout the weight-loss process and continue to add to it. It's a great way to keep yourself on track.

Q: What about having a few drinks now and then?

Having a few drinks conjures up images of relaxing at home or unwinding after a long day at work with good friends, good conversation, and good food. But then a drink or two becomes three or four—you reach for the pretzels and the peanuts—and suddenly your waistline is the only thing doing the unwinding. You can do everything right, but with just a few gulps, you might as well have been eating doughnuts all day. So be cautious. That said, depending on your plan, you can have an occasional drink on your meal plan; just make sure you balance those calories with food calories. Also be aware of the following:

- There are about 7 calories per gram of alcohol, compared with 4 calories per gram of carbohydrates or protein. (Fat has about 9 calories per gram.)
- Alcohol can lessen the body's ability to burn stored fat. Calories from alcohol are also likely to go right to your stomach—ever heard of a "beer belly"?
- Alcohol impairs a dieter's good judgment—which means you eat and drink more than you normally would. To top it off, most people enjoy eating

high-calorie, high-sodium snacks when they drink alcohol—three times the trouble if you're trying to lose weight.

- Alcohol can be especially harmful to dieters because blood sugar levels may drop more rapidly after having a drink. This drop in blood sugar can stimulate your appetite and disrupt your ability to tell when you've had enough to eat. Additionally, this can create fatigue, and your energy level will suffer.
- Alcohol interferes with the body's absorption of vitamins and minerals.
- Alcohol is often used as an inappropriate replacement for food, resulting in inadequate nutrition.

I'm not suggesting that you never drink again—in fact, moderate levels of alcohol consumption have been shown to reduce the chances of heart disease. But it is important to be conscious of what you consume. Simply having one beer a night adds more than 1,000 calories per week—that's an extra 15 pounds per year. A few glasses of wine over the course of one meal adds as much as 400 calories.

Beer. Twelve ounces of regular beer has about 150 calories; 12 ounces of light beer has 100 calories.

Wine. Five ounces of dry wine or champagne contains only 100 calories, which makes this a good choice—but watch out for sweet dessert wine, which has 226 calories.

Hard liquor. Just 1.5 ounces of 80 proof (40 percent alcohol) liquor is about 100 calories. Keep in mind that the higher the proof, the higher the calories. Remember, a typical serving of scotch on the rocks has about 1½ to 2 shots (depending on how well you know the bartender or if you're pouring the drink yourself). Also, be aware that the really sweet stuff such as schnapps (one shot) has 159 calories, and crème de menthe has 186 calories.

Mixed drinks. Alcohol itself is packed with calories, but when you add in mixers—soda, juice, sugar, and other ingredients—well, watch out. Turning rum into a rum and Coke nearly doubles the calories; the same goes for a gin and tonic. A suggestion: Keep it simple and on the rocks.

Obviously, the larger the drink, the higher the calorie content. If your favorite bar or restaurant serves bucket-size margaritas, you can easily drink more than 1,000 calories—without the chips and guacamole. Try to choose smaller drinks and avoid the creamy and frozen ones. And don't be shy—ask for diet sodas for all your mixers; it makes a difference of about 80 to 100 calories.

For the record:

- Bloody Mary (1.5 ounces vodka, 6 ounces tomato juice, dash of Tabasco and pepper) = 131 calories
- White wine spritzer (4 ounces white wine with club soda) = 80 calories
- Vodka and diet soda = 100 calories
- Piña colada (8 ounces) = 464 calories
- Long Island iced tea (8 ounces) = 227 calories
- Mudslide (1.5 ounces coffee liqueur, 1.5 ounces Irish cream, 1.5 ounces vodka) = 441 calories
- Margarita in a pint glass = 650 calories
- Martini (3 ounces) = 187 calories

And lastly, for comparison, two glazed Dunkin' Donuts has 360 calories.

Q: I travel frequently; how can I stay on track?

The key here is planning. For instance, you should request a refrigerator and microwave in your hotel room; most times you will not be charged any additional fees. Do a Google search for supermarkets or grocery stores in the area where you'll be staying and make a quick trip to buy foods that fit your plan. Soups, cereals, and some of the nonfrozen items might work best. Not all restaurants offer calorie information, but you can still try to keep a general idea of how many calories you're eating each day. I'm not suggesting counting calories, but you can keep most of your meals in check by using the many free Smartphone apps that are available.

Lastly, if you know you're traveling and eating a bit more, try increasing your exercise—perhaps even doubling it when you're away. Walking is always the best and easiest to implement.

For the Trip

Always try to plan the food part of your trip. You probably spend time planning all the other details, but you often neglect the food and fitness aspects. Just because you're going on vacation doesn't mean you have to take a break from making good health choices. Whether you're traveling by plane, train, car, or bus, you can pack a cooler or bag with food. But what to pack?

- **Cereal in a cup.** These are portion controlled at 1.5 ounces, and they're easy to store and easy to use. (Keep choices under 120 calories per ounce.)
- **Sandwiches.** Precut them so you can pull out portion-controlled sections at different times during the trip without making a mess. Try chicken, turkey, cheese, or peanut butter and jelly (on 100 percent whole wheat bread).
- **Water.** Dehydration can cause or exacerbate hunger and fatigue. (For plane travel, you need to purchase water after you go through security.)
- **Energy bars.** While they can be high in calories, they are often better than a slice of pizza or a candy bar.
- **Nonfat yogurt.** Yogurt is a great portable snack (although it is perishable). You can pack a 3-ounce container in an insulated bag or take a small cooler, but understand that this might be counted as one of your carry-on bags.
- **Nuts.** They're a good source of protein, and they help fend off hunger. Portion them into 1-ounce bags (about 160 calories each).
- **Dried or freeze-dried fruit.** Eat dried fruit in moderation; it's high in calories.
- **Fresh fruit.** Stick with fruits like apples and oranges that can withstand some rough treatment. Grapes or most any other fruit can be carried in a plastic container.

On the Road

Look for supermarkets. Go to www.google.com and put in the word "supermarket" and the ZIP code of the location. The names of local supermarkets will pop up on your screen.

Make fast food your friend. You can eat healthy fast food on the road. All you need to do is explore the Web sites of the various chains to get nutritional information beforehand and make the best picks.

Stay in health-minded motels/hotels. Call ahead or check online. Typically, newer properties have the latest exercise equipment and the best fitness facilities, but check around and ask to see photos. Many hotels such as Hyatt and Westin have made it their business to have fitness-friendly properties.

Upon Arrival

Scope out the territory. Find healthy restaurants and markets in the area. Search online or call the concierges or hotel managers of a few local hotels (even if you're not staying there) to ask for recommendations. Find out if the menu's available on the Internet so you can make decisions before you get there—it's always better to map out your food choices ahead of time.

Get moving. Ask if there are hiking or walking trails nearby, local fitness facilities, or other interesting activities that require you to move. If your motel or hotel has no gym, try the International Health, Racquet and Sportsclub Association (IHRSA) Passport Program, which gives members of participating IHRSA clubs guest privileges at more than 3,000 clubs worldwide. Locate a club by going to www.healthclubs.com/passport.

Visit a farmers' market. The USDA Web site www.ams.usda.gov/farmersmarkets/ provides information on places to find fresh, healthful food.

Get a kitchen. Find out if the place you're staying has rooms with kitchens, or, at the least, ask for a fridge in your room—even if you have to pay a small fee. That way, you can stock up on healthy fruits and veggies. Also, see if you can get a microwave—not that you should spend your vacation cooking in your room, but you can use it to make snacks like popcorn or even microwaveable packaged foods such as those at www.simplyasia.net or www.worldpantry.com (Annie Chun's foods).

Plan to Be Active

Get wet. Swimmers Guide is a free online database that contains a detailed international directory of "publicly accessible" swimming pools. The site proclaims that it lists "18,266 facilities with 19,443 full-size, year-round swimming pools in 10,398 cities and towns in 165 countries." Go to www.swimmersguide.com.

Get out and walk. Research shows that the more scenic your walks are, the more you'll want to take them. Walking burns 246 calories per hour. Again, go online and do a search at www.google.com or www.yahoo.com. Type in "walking tours," "hikes," and/or "bike rentals," and the location you'll be visiting.

Go sightseeing. Download tours to your MP3 player at www.audiosteps.com or www.tourcaster.com.

Give it the old college try. Visit nearby universities or colleges—typically a beautiful way to spend a morning or afternoon just walking around.

Go for a hike. Here are a few sites to visit:
- Trimbleoutdoors.com (http://backpacker.trimbleoutdoors.com/backpacker/home.aspx) offers thousands of day hikes and includes interactive maps, aerial and scenic photos, video, and downloadable GPS files.
- Localhikes.com (www.localhikes.com) provides details and reviews on bikes in and around metropolitan areas in the United States. Submitted by volunteer reporters..
- Trails.com (www.trails.com) charges $49.95 per year, but it does offer a 14-day free trial. The site offers detailed route descriptions, driving directions, guidebook-quality trail maps, photos, and ratings and reviews from its members for more than 38,000 trails.
- Recreation.gov (www.recreation.gov) is the US government's one-stop shop for the outdoors. There is information on everything from monuments, hiking, canoeing, kayaking, water-skiing, and rock climbing to wildlife observation and caving. It lists 388 National Park Service areas, 3,200 federal recreation areas, and 16,741 miles of trails in parks that range in size from one-fifth of an acre to 13.2 million acres.

Do yoga. Find a yoga class at www.yogafinder.com or do yoga with the help of your computer using www.yogatoday.com,which offers free daily classes online.

Hire a trainer or take a lesson or two. A great way to stay in shape is to hire a personal trainer. Once you make an appointment, there is a high likelihood that you'll show up (especially if you're committed to pay). Look for trainers certified by the American College of Sports Medicine (www.acsm.org), the National Strength and Conditioning Association (www.nsca-lift.org,) or the American Council on Exercise (www.acefitness.org). You can also take lessons in activities such as tennis, yoga, volleyball, or horseback riding.

Here are a few other activities to explore:
(Calorie expenditures is based on a 155-pound person.)

- Bicycling. Burn 422 to 562 calories per hour.
- Kayaking. Burn 352 calories per hour.
- Horseback riding. Burn 281 calories per hour.
- Canoeing. Burn 281 calories per hour.
- Water-skiing. Burn 422 calories per hour.

What to Pack

- Fitness DVDs. Join www.netflix.com or buy them at www.amazon.com.
- Fitness cards. If you don't want to sit in your hotel room watching a fitness DVD, try the wonderful and handy fitness travel cards by Sane Fit (www.sanefit.com) or Training Fan (www.trainingfan.com) (i.e., yoga fan and training fan)—they're both great.

Q: How can I prepare for times when I feel overwhelmed (like when I'm out with friends)?

Despite our best intentions, when it comes to weight loss and healthy habits, we all have our weak moments—those times when it seems we always slip up, no matter how determined we are. Your weakness might be eating at restaurants, snacking at work, or overeating when you're under stress. How can you combat these uncomfortable eating situations?

Well, the Olympics got me thinking about what we can learn from elite athletes—how do they overcome their moments of adversity? What I found was that almost all world-class athletes practice mental rehearsal. Haven't you ever heard the expression "Practice makes perfect"? The concept is to rehearse an upcoming event, but not on the field—in your mind. "You're using imagery to trick your brain into having an experience you didn't actually have," says Shane Murphy, PhD, a professor of psychology at Western Connecticut State University and former sports psychologist to the US Olympic team.

Skiers imagine each run down the slope, perfectly executing every turn in order to "train" their bodies to do the same when they actually compete. Rumor has it that Jack Nicklaus, the great golfer, never missed a putt in his mind—he would never take a shot without using imagery before hitting the ball. "For an athlete, it's like having an instant 'preplay'—seeing the event and practicing (including fixing mistakes), all before it happens—to avoid making the big mistakes on the field," says Jim Afremow, PhD, a sports physiologist at the Athletes' Performance Center in Tempe, Arizona.

And mental rehearsal is not just for athletes. According to the *American Journal of Surgery,* surgeons who practice their skills using mental rehearsal perform better in the operating room.

So why not use those same techniques to show yourself what it will feel like to be free of a particular overeating shackle—such as mindlessly munching your way through an entire row of Oreos to relieve the pressure of a bad day at work?

Roadblock Anticipation

You don't have to physically practice standing in the buffet line at your best friend's wedding in order to learn how to turn down fattening food. Instead, you can rehearse the scenario in your mind so that, rather than eating the triple-layer chocolate supreme cake with a scoop of ice cream on the side, you can revise the ending.

"We train athletes to anticipate their reaction to negative situations, so they are able to create a positive outcome. For instance, a skater falling in midsession, a soccer player playing in inclement weather, or a sprinter competing against a world record holder—the athlete needs to know how he is going to respond in advance. The same applies to avoiding potential diet disasters," says Murphy.

Confidence Building

Athletes and nonathletes alike are faced with uncomfortable issues, and in order to break away from the anticipated fear or anxiety of an event, you need to build confidence. And what builds that confidence? The experience of doing it right. In this way, mental rehearsal helps athletes overcome performance anxiety. For example, maybe the holidays make you anxious. You already know what to expect next Thanksgiving, so you can mentally rehearse saying no to the stuffing, gravy, and candied sweet potatoes, and see your plate filled with plain turkey and vegetables and other, less fattening "trimmings." As Louis Pasteur said, "Chance favors the prepared mind."

Q: I have no willpower—can I still lose weight?

You need to use *power,* not willpower. People often wonder if they have enough willpower to actually make the behavior change.

The fact is, research has shown that we have a limited amount of self-control or willpower. Mark Muraven and Roy F. Baumeister, reporting in the journal *Psychological Bulletin,* found "evidence that self-control may consume a limited resource. Exerting self-control may consume self-control strength, reducing the amount of strength available for subsequent self-control efforts." Think of using willpower as working your muscles—meaning it can be exhausted and fail if used too much. There's also been evidence to show that even watching others use willpower can exhaust your own willpower. Additionally, research at Florida State University found that acts of self-control deplete relatively large amounts of glucose. And self-control failures are more likely to occur when glucose is low or cannot be mobilized effectively to the brain. Willpower has been called a "glucose guzzler"—sapping you of much-needed energy.

Do you really believe that all you need is good healthy dose of drawing the line in the sand to break the patterns you've been living by? Look, I'm not going to sit here and tell you that there isn't some self-control or willpower involved in weight control, but it's significantly less than you think.

Seriously. Weight loss is more about power than willpower. You need to give yourself the power to lose weight. The point is not to get discouraged because you think you lack the willpower or discipline to lose weight—that's not what's going to help you lose and keep the weight off.

What will work? Preparation, personal detective work, and being realistic and honest with yourself and your behaviors.

Are You Really "Willing" It to Happen, or Is It All in Your Mind?

Harvard researcher and scientist Daniel M. Wegner argues that conscious will means you're in control and actually doing something to affect an outcome. In other words, you are causing the results by your actions. For instance, exercising more, resisting the cake, and eating healthier foods result in your losing weight. According to Wegner's writings in *The Illusion of Conscious Will,* the feeling that we are simply exerting willpower in order to do these things may not be a true reading of what is happening in our minds and bodies as our actions are produced. Is it really nothing more than your simply resisting temptation? Or is changing a behavior more about doing the prep work that sets you up to succeed?

It's Magic

Think about a magician—when you see a magician performing his or her illusion, it's seamless. You don't "see" how the magic works—it just works. But the reality (just like losing and controlling your weight) is much more complicated. The magician did not just come on stage and perform the illusion. He or she worked hard, doing research, creating or buying proper equipment, developing a performance technique, then practicing, evaluating, reformatting, and practicing more.

Losing and controlling weight appears to be just about willpower—willing something to take place—but really it's about preparation, practice, failure, planning, and so on. Weight loss is more about power than about willpower. You need to give yourself the power to lose weight.

Wegner continues in his writings: "The real causal sequence underlying human behavior involves a massively complicated set of mechanisms. . . . Each of our actions is really the culmination of an intricate set of physical and mental processes, including psychological mechanisms that correspond to the traditional concept of will in that they involve linkages between our thoughts and our actions."

What You Should Do

The point is to not get discouraged because you think you lack the willpower or discipline to lose weight—that's not what's going to get you through this process.

Weight loss or control is not as simple as willing yourself not to eat that cookie. That's not what's going to help you lose and keep the weight off. What will work:

preparation, personal diet detective work, and being realistic and honest with yourself about your behaviors. Using mental rehearsal—that is, thinking in advance about uncomfortable eating situations and creating an if/then plan for how you're going to overcome them, figuring out what you will eat instead of the high-calorie cookie, making sure the types of foods you want to avoid are not even in your sight—these are just some of the techniques that will help you to create power and give you the ability to practice so-called self-control.

Last, but certainly not least, understanding the concept of creating automatic behaviors helps to create power. As I've said time and time again, it's just too difficult to think constantly about dieting—it will not work. Successful maintainers have figured out ways to make their behaviors and choices second nature.

Activities like setting your alarm clock at night, putting on your shoes before leaving the house, and remembering how to drive to work do not require much thought. The idea is to apply the same principles to your diet. Arrange your personal environment so it maximizes your chances of losing weight and maintaining your loss and minimizes your chances of slipping up. Avoid cues that tempt you. If you drive by Dunkin' Donuts on the way to work and can't resist stopping for a box of doughnuts, change your route. Don't leave foods in the house that are going to "set you off"—or at least put them out of reach. Make exercise something you have to do in order to complete another daily task (walking a child to school, biking to work, etc.).

Again, my goal here is to give you a better understanding of why mere willpower, a resolve to eat healthy (not eat the "bad" stuff) and/or to exercise more, probably will not cut it for weight control. Instead, direct that "willpower" energy into something that will make a difference: planning, practice, education, etc. It will be worth it.

A Final Word

Now that you've learned a way to control calories, it's also important to slowly integrate more fitness and healthier, more nutritious eating into your diet. Make sure to read my column each week on www.DietDetective.com and also keep up with me on my Facebook page, www.Facebook.com/DietDetective, or on Twitter, www.Twitter.com/DietDetective.

ABOUT THE AUTHOR

Charles Platkin, Phd, JD, MPH, aka the Diet Detective, is one of the country's leading nutrition and public health advocates. His syndicated health, nutrition, and fitness column, "Diet Detective," appears in more than 100 media outlets. Platkin is also the founder of DietDetective.com (an Everyday Health/Waterfront Media License), which offers nutrition, food, and fitness information along with a weight-loss program providing customizable meal plans and fitness regimens that put his wellness principles into action. Additionally, Platkin is an assistant professor (visiting) at the CUNY School of Public Health in New York City. He was the host of WE TV's series *I Want to Save Your Life.*

Platkin has been quoted as a health expert in thousands of publications, including *USA Today*, the *Los Angeles Times,* the *New York Times,* the *New York Post,* the *New York Daily News, Newsday,* the *Chicago Tribune, Oprah, Time, Newsweek, Ladies Home Journal, Men's Health, Shape, Self,* and *Fitness.* He has also appeared on *Today, Good Morning America, Nightline, The Early Show,* National Public Radio, CNN, CNBC, BBC America, and others.

He is a member of the American Society for Nutritional Sciences, the American Obesity Association, Society for Public Health Education, Society for Nutrition Education, the American Public Health Association, Sigma Xi (Scientific Research Society), the Delta Omega Honorary Society in Public Health, and the American Council on Exercise. He received his undergraduate degree from Cornell University, a law degree from Fordham University, a Master's of Public Health from Florida International University, and a PhD in Public Health from Florida International University. He is also an ACE certified personal trainer.

Platkin is the author of five books. His first book, *Breaking the Pattern,* was a bestseller in hardcover and has been used by addiction clinics to assist patients with resolving drug and alcohol-related issues and by more than 20 universities around the country as a text to teach behavioral change techniques to nutrition and dietetic counseling students. His latest books are *The Diet Detective's Count Down* (Simon and Schuster, 2007) and *The Diet Detective's Calorie Bargain Bible* (Simon and Schuster, 2008).

PHOTO CREDITS

Thanks to our team for a successful photo shoot in which we captured the majority of the food images for *The Diet Detective's All-American Diet*. Special thanks to director Sonia Molinari, project manager Mary Cummings, Alex Pereira, and the fabulous Micah Molinari; senior photographers Francisco Aguila and Jeremy Merriam; and photographer Kerri Brewer, to whom all photo credits are due, other than those provided by the companies; senior food stylist Catherine Hoffman; and our assistants Bev Chin, Will Boone, Jonathan Friedman, and Kyle Broder.

The following companies provided images and releases for those images. Please note that simply because a company is listed below doesn't mean that all of the product images in the book were provided by that company; many were shot by our team.

ACKNOWLEDGMENTS

This book has been a longtime passion, and I have many people to thank for helping me to finally bring it to fruition.

First, I would like to thank Shira Isenberg, RD, for her dedication and unyielding commitment to getting this book in working order. She is just amazing. Next, Sonia Riahi, who has helped me with my TV show, my PhD research, and now this wonderful book. She is also simply amazing. Judy Kern, who is the world's fastest and best editor—a real find. I hope she never retires or gets tired of reading my "stuff." Also, this book would not be organized, logical, or readable without the help of Mary Cummings. I'm a huge fan of Shira, Sonia, Judy, and Mary.

I would like to thank my literary agent, friend, and partner, Scott Waxman, for believing in the idea from the start and pushing to make this book a reality. Scott, you are truly the best salesperson when you believe—and you believed.

Thanks to Shannon Welch, who also believed in the concept—and "got" the idea quickly without any "selling" required; and to C. Linda Dingler for helping to design the information so that readers see what is meant to be seen in order for them to make clear, precise decisions, and for being a calming force in a complicated process. Last of all, Alex Pereira, who helps deal with and fix all the little problems that can ruin your day.

Index

Underscored page references denote boxed text.